Handbook of
Community
Health

Handbook of Community Health/ Y 1 0 5

MURRAY GRANT, M.D., D.P.H:

Chief Medical Advisor to the U.S. General Accounting Office

Former Director of Public Health for the District of Columbia

Former Clinical Professor of Community Health, George Washington University School of Medicine, Washington, D.C.

Former Clinical Professor of Public Health, Department of Preventive Medicine and Public Health, Howard University College of Medicine, Washington, D.C.

THIRD EDITION

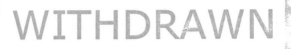

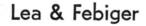

Lea & Febiger   Philadelphia • 1981

Lea & Febiger
600 S. Washington Square
Philadelphia, PA 19106

Library of Congress Cataloging in Publication Data

Grant, Murray, 1926–
    Handbook of community health.

    Includes bibliographies and index.
    1. Public health. 2. Medicine, Preventive. I. Title.
[DNLM: 1. Preventive medicine. 2. Public health. Wa 100
G762h]
RA425.G68   1981   614   80-26182
ISBN 0-8121-0760-8

FIRST EDITION, 1967
    Reprinted, 1969
    Reprinted, 1973
SECOND EDITION, 1975
    Reprinted, 1976
    Reprinted, 1979
THIRD EDITION, 1981

Published in Great Britain by Henry Kimpton Publishers, London

PRINTED IN THE UNITED STATES OF AMERICA

Print No. 3 2 1

Preface

It is unlikely that 14 years ago, at the time of publication of the first edition, one could have been so bold as to have predicted the extent to which government, particularly the Federal establishment, would have played such a pre-eminent role in the health affairs of every man, woman and child in the country in just a few years. This edition, by updating existing chapters and incorporating several new chapters, has attempted to recognize these salient facts and to discuss the growing Federal role in many areas of health.

While this clearly represents the most dramatic change of the past decade in the public health arena, others must also be recognized. Accordingly, a new chapter on geriatrics has attempted to place this growing field in perspective, and one on medical sociology is included to place emphasis on an area that continues to develop. The important role played by government sponsored professional standards review organizations and health systems agencies is reflected in the chapters discussing quality of care and health planning. The issues which confront us in the health manpower field are also outlined in a separate chapter in which some

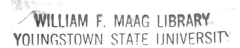

v

emphasis has been placed on the important role played by different health professionals in addition to physicians. One of the most widely discussed health topics today, health care delivery, also receives separate attention.

This book remains, as was the intent of the first edition, not as a comprehensive text, but as an introduction to the field, designed for those who need or desire to learn something about the content of community health and hopefully whetting the appetite of some to subsequently explore in further depth.

MURRAY GRANT

Washington, D.C.

Contents

Contents

Chapter 1

Fundamentals of Epidemiology and Genetics

EPIDEMIOLOGY

Epidemiologic principles were, for many years, employed exclusively for the study and control of communicable diseases. Experience has taught us, however, that the techniques used in studying communicable diseases have a much wider applicability throughout the fields of general medicine and public health.

Concept of an Epidemic

In the past, the term "epidemic" was used to describe an outbreak of infectious disease. Current definitions use "excessive prevalence." This characteristic is exemplified by many non-infectious diseases, for example, atherosclerosis and lung cancer.

Sometimes the existence of an epidemic is serious, particularly when it involves a large number of persons and occurs over a short period of time. In contrast, the risk to an American dying from coronary heart disease is now every bit as high as the risk of death experienced during past major epidemics of infectious disease; the

1

slow growth of the epidemic has, however, concealed its size.

Understanding the Causation of Disease

The primary purpose of epidemiology is to acquire knowledge of causal mechanisms that can form a basis for the development of preventive measures. To accomplish this one must:

1. Develop hypotheses that explain patterns of disease distribution.
2. Test those hypotheses through specifically designed studies.
3. Test the validity of the concept on which control programs are based through the collection and analysis of epidemiologic data.
4. Classify all persons into groups which appear to have common etiological factors.

The Purpose of Epidemiology

Epidemiology may be broadly defined as the study of the distribution of a disease or condition in a population and of the various factors that influence this distribution. Whereas in the clinical practice of medicine the focus is on the individual patient, in epidemiology the focus is on the group. Large numbers of people are considered in reference to a specific disease in terms of age, sex, race, heredity, occupation and other characteristics. While the private physician concerns himself with his patient, the epidemiologist must view the whole population. By an epidemiologic approach the course of a disease is described and its various characteristics are defined, the cause may be established, its usual symptoms described and its prognosis predicted. Epidemiologic studies provide information on the occurrence and distribution of disease and collect data which may be useful in instituting control measures.

It is important to know how the duration of a disease and the probability of possible outcomes such as recovery or death vary by age, sex, geography, etc. This information can be used not only for prognostic purposes, but also to stimulate hypotheses concerning the specific factors which may be directly involved in detecting the course of the disease.

Forming a Hypothesis

An epidemiologic hypothesis should provide information on:
1. The characteristics of those individuals to whom the hypothesis applies.
2. The cause being considered.
3. The expected effect.
4. The dose-response relationship.
5. The time-response relationship.

It should be noted that almost any set of observations will be compatible with more than one hypothesis. It is necessary, therefore, to select the one that appears worthy of testing.

Major uses of epidemiology are:
1. To analyze the respective role of agent, host and environment in the development and natural history of disease.
2. To analyze the occurrence and distribution of disease according to characteristics such as age, sex, race, occupation and heredity.
3. To study, outline and define problems of health and disease by analysis of incidence, prevalence and mortality.
4. To help complete the clinical picture and natural history of disease by group analyses.

5. To estimate a person's risk of developing a disease and his chances for survival.
6. To search for factors related to health and disease by observation of group customs and habits.
7. To evaluate the need for and effectiveness of health services through field studies.

Agent, Host and Environment

The epidemiologist undertakes studies of the agent's characteristics and relationship to the disease under observation. Snow's epidemiologic studies, which clearly demonstrated the relationship of the development of cholera to drinking water, provide an excellent example of the epidemiologist at work.

The epidemiologist studies the interaction between agent and host and concerns himself with the susceptibility or resistance of the host. This, in turn, may be influenced by factors such as heredity, age, sex or race or by induced immunity resulting from immunization programs.

The epidemiologist's interest in the environment as it relates to disease includes factors such as temperature and humidity as well as socioeconomic conditions, housing and occupational conditions, general levels of sanitation and even a population's literacy.

Agent. Agents of disease may be physical, chemical or biologic. Physical agents may be mechanical, thermal, or radiant. The motor vehicle is a common example of a mechanical agent. Thermal agents may cause extreme cold or heat, either of which is harmful to the human body. The chief radiant agent is x ray, but atomic radiation (fallout) constitutes another type of radiant agent.

Chemical agents may produce illness by direct contact or by ingestion or inhalation. Carbon monoxide is a good example of an inhalation agent. Food poisoning outbreaks may occur as a result of contamination of food with fluoride. Various nutritional disturbances may occur as a result of deficiency or overabundance of certain elements in the diet.

Biologic agents include worms and insects, protozoa, fungi, bacteria and viruses. These play an extremely important role in the causation of disease.

Host. Many factors influence the susceptibility of the host to injury by an agent. For example, customs and habits may play a role; certain religious groups, for instance, are forbidden to eat pork and therefore will not develop trichinosis. On the other hand, brucellosis is rare in countries where milk consumption is low.

The body has a variety of defense mechanisms. The front line of defense includes the skin, hair and nails. There are a variety of physiologic defense mechanisms, for example, the cough reflex, the ability of the liver to detoxify chemicals or of the bones to store certain metals and the body's heat-regulatory mechanism. Lastly, the body may have or develop immunity.

There are, moreover, other more general factors involved. These include age, sex and color. Some diseases affect certain age groups or one sex or color more than others. The host's heredity is important as may be his previous experience with a specific agent.

Environment. The environment may be favorable to the host or to the agent, and changes in the environment may have a profound effect by shifting the balance from one to the other. The location of a community on land that may be fertile, near water, unproductive or far from a water supply will determine the ability of flora and fauna to grow and multiply. Climate and seasonal factors may determine whether a particular insect vector can survive. The Arctic, for example, is too cold for mosquitoes; malaria, therefore does not occur there.

The level of sanitation, including provision for a potable water supply and proper methods of sewage disposal, is an important factor. The biologic environment is of great importance. A community that has a good rat-eradication program would not expect much in the way of murine typhus.

Measures of Disease Frequency

Incidence is the number of cases of the disease which occur during a specified period of time. The incidence rate is this number per specified unit of population.

Attack rate is an incidence rate applied when a population is at risk for a limited period of time; for example, if there were an outbreak of scarlet fever in a school with a population of 1,000, and 120 children developed the disease, the attack rate would be 12%.

Prevalence is the frequency of a disease at a designated point in time and the prevalence rate is the proportion of the population which exhibits the disease at that time.

In studying a disease, the epidemiologist must examine incubation periods, the extent of communicability, possible sources of infection and methods of transmission. He must also ascertain the usual prevalence of the disease. This requires a review of case reports in the event of a disease required by law to be reported, but more often than not it will require a more intensive investigation, including consultation with private physicians or hospitals or even random sampling of households. Seasonal or cyclic variations must be studied, including the peculiar prevalence of a disease at certain times of the year or even at periodic intervals. Automobile accidents, for example, tend to be most common in the late fall.

Mortality studies are much more simple to carry out than are those concerned with morbidity. Precise data on the latter are difficult to secure and also require substantial effort on the part of the investigator. Mortality data, on the other hand, are usually readily available from a review of death certificates. It is primarily for this reason that such extensive use has been made of these materials.

The Clinical Picture of Disease

Every medical student experiences difficulty in finding the patient whose symptoms exactly fit the classic textbook picture, because typical textbook descriptions result from group analysis of signs and symptoms. This, again, is the field of the epidemiologist. For example, a study of a series of cases of coronary thrombosis will indicate the most common features and the natural history of events. This requires, however, a detailed study together with careful examination of laboratory material and close attention to long-term follow-up of the patients.

A similar study is required to estimate the person's risk of developing a disease and his chances for survival. Careful attention, however, must be paid to the person's existing health status. It is clear, for example, that an aged person already suffering from chronic respiratory disease is more likely to succumb during an epidemic of influenza than is a vigorous, healthy adolescent. Pregnancy, too, may have a marked effect upon risk and survival.

Habits and Customs

Habits relating to the consumption of certain foods, cooking processes, cleanliness and handling of food and milk all contribute to the occurrence and distribution of disease. Similarly, carelessness in the home may result in accidental injury or death from falls or poisoning. Social customs relating to the disposal of excreta or to attitudes towards sex or promiscuity obviously may have an impact upon the occurrence of disease.

Health Services and Control Measures

A study of accidents in a community should reveal in what age group accidental deaths tend to occur and from what causes. It should also indicate the most common sites at which they occur. Such a study may point to ways in which a health program may contribute to the possible reduction of these accidental deaths. Similarly, a detailed study of the health status of a sampling of school-aged children in a community may reveal obvious deficiencies, such as finding many children with visual, hearing or emotional defects. Again, this may point to the need for the development of a community program aimed at improving the existing situation.

On the other hand, consider a community which has, for many years, had a fairly comprehensive immunization program in effect against diphtheria. An epidemiologic study in that community may reveal a low level of immunity to diphtheria, particularly in low-income areas, thus pointing to deficiencies in the existing program and defining ways by which the situation may be improved.

An outbreak of disease in a community should, of course, be followed immediately by appropriate control measures. This will usually necessitate a detailed epidemiologic investigation of the outbreak in which data are gathered concerning the prevalence, characteristics, symptomatology, course and prognosis of the disease. It may also, however, serve to initiate control meaures, such as the tracing, immunization or quarantine of contacts.

Epidemiologic Study Methods

There are three general kinds of epidemiologic studies: retrospective, prospective and experimental.

Retrospective Studies. Under this procedure, *already available* records are scrutinized. A group with the disease under study is selected, together with an appropriate control group, and their characteristics are compared.

Prospective Studies. Under this procedure, *records are developed* from a study of a population. One group with the disease or characteristic is defined and studied, together with an appropriate control group which does not have this disease or characteristic.

While prospective studies have many advantages over the retrospective type, they are generally more difficult and time-consuming to pursue. In the latter, records are already available for analysis, while in the former they must be created from a study of a population yet to be designed.

Experimental Studies. A more certain way of developing epidemiologic facts is by properly designed experimental studies. One of the best examples of this kind of study is afforded by the comparison of the effect on teeth of fluoridated water with that of water having little fluoride content. Such a study was begun in the state of New York during 1945, in the cities of Newburgh and Kingston. Sodium fluoride was added to the water supply of Newburgh and the dental status of children in this city was compared for several years with that of children in Kingston where no sodium fluoride was added to the water supply.

Clearly, experimental studies offer the best type of epidemiologic study; the design requirements are, however, stringent, and the amount of time, effort and money required make this kind of study much more difficult to initiate and carry through than either retrospective or prospective studies.

Examples of Epidemiologic Studies

Example No. 1. On September 25, 1944, a report was received by the New York City Health Department that 11 men had been admitted to a hospital in the city suffering from cyanosis and shock. The health department's investigation revealed that all had become ill between 7:00 and 10:00 that morning, within 5 to 30 minutes following breakfast which all had eaten in the same cafeteria. The men were aged between 60 and 80, and all were derelicts who lived in cheap rooming houses in the Bowery.

The clinical picture was similar in all. They became dizzy, felt weak and complained of abdominal cramps. All had diarrhea, 8 vomited; 4 became unconscious. They were admitted to the hospital by ambulance. Blood counts and urine examinations revealed no abnormality. The men were treated for shock and also received gastric lavage. All but one, the oldest, recovered. The oldest man died the next morning; autopsy revealed bronchopneumonia and a diffuse brown discoloration of the organs.

In view of the cyanosis, specimens of blood were examined spectroscopically for evidence of methemoglobin. Clear evidence of its presence was found in each patient. All the men denied use of drugs prior to their illness.

The cafeteria in which they had eaten was then checked. It had generally low standards of sanitation and was located in a poor section of town. All but one of the men had eaten oatmeal, rolls and coffee; one ate oatmeal only. Therefore, close attention was directed to this food. The oatmeal had been purchased in 5-pound paper cartons; water and salt had been added, the mixture stirred and allowed to boil. Altogether, 125 persons had been served that morning; yet apparently only 11 had become sick. The water came from the city water supply. The salt used for cooking was kept in a can near the stove. On observing this material it was noticed to have a faint yellow color. The cook stated that he filled this can from a supply kept on the shelf. When this shelf was examined, two containers were found; one of these was clearly filled with salt; the other was filled with a yellowish powder. This powder was later determined to be saltpeter, which the owner used in curing meat. Both containers were examined in the health department laboratory. The yellowish powder was found to contain 92% sodium nitrite. It became clear, now, that this material had been used in mistake for salt, since the symptoms exhibited by the men were referable to and certainly compatible with sodium nitrite poisoning.

The question remained as to why only 11 of 125 persons who consumed the oatmeal had become sick. Inquiry did not reveal the existence of any additional cases. A subsequent examination of the cafeteria's salt-shakers showed that several of these also contained sodium nitrite. It now seemed evident that these salt-shakers were the important factor involved. Some men added no salt to their oatmeal; only a few had used those saltshakers containing the sodium nitrite. Incidentally, subsequent examination of the patient's blood revealed the presence of nitrites.

Example No. 2. A study was made of all cases of poliomyelitis that occurred in New York City in 1949 and 1950, in order to compare the epidemiologic features of the disease in infants under 1 year with those in children and adults. There were 2,446 cases and 198 deaths in 1949, while in 1950, there were 1,064 cases and 64 deaths. Approximately 58% of the cases occurred among males and 42% among females. Ninety-two of the patients (2.6%) were infants under 1 year of age. Diagnosis was made on a clinical basis using any three of the following criteria—acute onset, fever, rigidity of the neck or spasm, flaccid paralysis, elevation of spinal fluid protein and more than 10 cells per mm in the spinal fluid. Approximately 90% of the patients were hospitalized.

The attack rate was found to be highest in infants from 6 months to 1 year of age. This was also true of the case fatality rate. The lowest percentage of those paralyzed was found in the group comprised of children between the ages of 5 and 15 years. All patients in the first 3 months of life were paralyzed; 90% of infants were paralyzed as compared to about 66% in all other age groups. These significant differences could only be determined, however, by a careful analysis of the data presented above.

These two examples of epidemiologic studies are described merely to indicate the method of approach used. The two entirely different problems also indicate the variety of problem areas which are subject to this type of investigation.

GENETICS

In considering the causative factors in the production of disease a question frequently raised is, "Which is more important, heredity or environment?" The question of environment is discussed in several chapters of this book. A brief, if elementary, discussion of heredity is therefore in order.

Fundamentals of Genetics

Sexual reproduction involves the conjugation of two germ cells and union of their nuclei. In the formation of the germ cells, the ovum and spermatozoon nuclei undergo a special type of division called "reduction division" or "meiosis." In this process, the normal number of 46 chromosomes in each cell is reduced by half. The act of fertilization then restores the chromosome number to 46. A human being, therefore, possesses 23 pairs of chromosomes, one chromosome of each pair coming from the father and the other from the mother. During the subsequent growth and development of the fertilized egg, the number of chromosomes is maintained at 46 by the process of mitosis, or "regular" cell division.

Any deviation in these processes of meiosis and mitosis may lead to abnormalities. For example, a final chromosome count of 47 rather than 46 is usually associated with Down's syndrome (mongolism). This abnormality is particularly prone to occur in children whose mothers were past the age of 35 years when the children were born. One immediately can see a place for genetic counselling under these circumstances.

The two sets of 23 chromosomes that an individual possesses (one from each parent) differ considerably in their morphology, and many of the chromosomes are distinguishable from each other. Genes are the basic unit of heredity and are concerned with the determination of a specific trait. They are arranged in a linear manner along the length of the chromosome, and it has been estimated that there are approximately 10,000 genes in the human chromosome set. There are two genes for each inherited trait, one from the mother and the other from the father. A mutation is a basic change in a gene which produces an effect different from what is normally expected.

The corresponding genes from each parent are called alleles and control the same hereditary characteristic. A pair of defective genes may produce an abnormality. At the present time, most abnormal hereditary conditions cannot be proven to result exclusively from a single defective gene. During the process of meiosis there is a reshuffling of the parents' genes, thus explaining why children from the same parents have differing genotypes.

Mechanism of Heredity. An allele may be dominant or recessive. A trait carried by a dominant allele is always manifest in the person possessing it. If both alleles in the gene-pair (one from each parent) are the same, the person is said to be homozygous. If the alleles are different, the person is said to be heterozygous. When the presence of a single gene at a specific locus produces an effect on the trait, this is called dominant inheritance. The family history in such cases will usually show direct transmission of the trait from parent to child, with 50% of the offspring being similarly affected, without regard to sex.

In recessive inheritance, both genes at a specific locus must be similar to produce the effect. Each parent of an affected child carries one gene for the trait but shows no clinical signs of the trait. The two carrier parents have a 25% chance of producing an affected child with each pregnancy.

The third type of inheritance is called sex-linked inheritance. This involves a transmission of traits by genes located on the two sex chromosomes, XX (female) and XY (male). Most of the sex-linked traits are transmitted by the X chromosomes. In females, the presence of one gene is usually masked by the normal gene on the second X chromosome. Since males have only one X chromosome, the presence of a single gene for the abnormal trait is sufficient to produce the clinical effect. Therefore, 50% of the male offspring of a female carrier would be affected. Hemophilia is a good example of a sex-linked recessive trait.

Use of Genetics in Preventive Medicine

Some diseases are due exclusively to genetic factors; examples are hemophilia, sickle cell anemia, fibrocystic disease of the pancreas and multiple polyposis of the colon. In other diseases, genetic factors appear to exert an important influence. Examples of this group include deaf-mutism, cataracts and Parkinsonism. Finally, there are many diseases in which genetic factors appear to exercise some influence, although the exact extent to which this is important is not known. Examples include cancer of the breast, gout, atherosclerosis, coronary artery disease, pernicious anemia, rheumatic fever, diabetes, epilepsy and asthma. Obviously, this last group includes many of the most important diseases known to afflict mankind. There are, of course, many other diseases which do not appear to be related in any way to genetic factors. Examples include conditions such as measles and pneumonia.

Knowledge of genetic factors may provide opportunities for primary prevention. A good example is the knowledge of blood groups in the use of transfusions, or of the Rh factor. Obviously, knowledge of the genetic factors involved in conditions such as diabetes or senile glaucoma should lead to examination of relatives of persons having these diseases, aimed at early detection and treatment to prevent unnecessary disability. In other conditions, such as in retinitis pigmentosa, genetic counselling pertaining to the parents' chances of begetting offspring with serious defects may result in voluntary abstinence from parenthood. Genetic counselling, during which an estimate of the risk is given to the involved parties, is becoming increasingly important in the health field today, as our knowledge of this subject continues to increase.

REFERENCES

Ast, D. B., and Schlesinger, E. R.: The conclusion of a ten-year study of water fluoridation, Amer. Jour. Publ. Health 46:265, 1956.

Barker, D. J. P.: *Practical Epidemiology,* Churchill-Livingston, New York, 1976.

Friedman, G. D.: *Primer of Epidemiology,* McGraw-Hill Book Co. Inc., New York, 1974.

Leavell, H. R., and Clark, E. G.: *Preventive Medicine for the Doctor in his Community,* 3rd Ed., New York, McGraw-Hill Book Co., Inc., 1958.

MacMahon, B, & Pugh, T. F.: *Epidemiology—Principles and Methods,* Little Brown & Co., Boston, 1970.

Morris, J. N.: *Uses of Epidemiology,* 3rd Ed., Edinburgh, E. and S. Livingstone, Ltd., 1972.

Rogers, Fred B.: *Studies in Epidemiology,* Selected Papers of Morris Greenberg, M. D., New York, G. P. Putnam Sons, 1965.

Schact, L. C.: *Human Genetics in Public Health,* Minneapolis, University of Minnesota Press, August, 1964.

Smillie, W. G., and Kilbourne, E. D.: *Human Heredity and Genetic Determinants of Disease, Preventive Medicine and Public Health,* 3rd Ed. New York, The Macmillan Co., 1963.

Chapter 2

Health Statistics

In his Presidential Address to the Section of Experimental Medicine and Therapeutics of the Royal Society of Medicine delivered in 1949, Professor G. W. Pickering made the following statement, "Therapeutics is the branch of medicine that, by its very nature, should be experimental. For if we take a patient afflicted with a malady, and we alter his condition of life, either by dieting him or by putting him to bed or by administering to him a drug, or by performing on him an operation, we are performing an experiment. And if we are scientifically inclined, we should record the results. Before concluding that a change for the better or for worse in the patient is due to the specific treatment employed, we must ascertain whether the result can be reported a significant number of times in similar patients, whether the result was merely due to the medical history of the disease, or, in other words, to the lapse of time, or whether it was due to some other factor which was necessarily associated with the therapeutic issue in question.

"This would seem the procedure to be expected of men with six years of scientific training behind them. But it has not been followed. Had it been done we should have gained a fairly precise knowledge of the place of individual methods of therapy in disease and our efficacy as doctors would have been enormously enhanced."

Need for and Use of Statistical Material

Those responsible for developing community health services have many needs for statistical data and a wide variety of uses for these materials. In addition to the public health worker's need for birth, death and morbidity data with which to compile various indices from which he can make certain inferences concerning the success or failure of the community's health activities, he can also use this material as indicative of the need for or lack of requirements for the development of a particular health program. In addition, he must acquire a body of statistical material with which he can evaluate cost of these programs and, in some cases, to justify the expenditure of public funds.

Statistics have been aptly described as "the eyes and ears of the public health worker." The public health officer who is without population and related demographic data concerning the community in which he works is really working in the dark. These statistics may reveal a high infant mortality in one area, an unusually high incidence of tuberculosis in another. On the other hand, they may reveal that maternal mortality is not a problem. If, for example, the health officer observes a reduction in birth rate in his community, he would immediately ask certain questions. Is this reduction due to a population age change, or is it the result of a family-planning program? What effect will this reduction have on the community's need for obstetric and pediatric facilities?

In order for the student to interpret properly the

many health-related articles in the literature, he must possess at least some basic knowledge and understanding of the principles of statistical methods. The student of epidemiology will also need to acquire some knowledge of statistics. Oftentimes, articles that purport to reveal new or otherwise significant results may be subject to serious question. To review these articles, however, the student should be able to use basic statistical methods in order to analyze the apparent results. Failing this, he is apt to accept the statements of others too readily and without desirable critical appraisal. Frequently, papers appear to imply the acceptance of data as being factual when, in reality, these "facts" may be mere hypotheses. The student must learn to distinguish carefully between what is hypothesis and what has clearly been shown to be factual. He should also be able to understand clearly the meaning, significance and validity of the various tables, charts and graphs used in medical literature today. In Francis Bacon's words, "Read not to contradict and confute; nor to believe and take for granted; nor to find talk and discourse; but to weigh and consider."

Source of Vital Statistics

The collection, recording and interpretation of vital statistics have, for many years, been recognized as an important governmental responsibility.

The Census. In the United States, a national census is taken every 10 years; the last was carried out in 1980. The census provides not only a simple listing of all persons in the United States, but also the geographic location, age distribution, sex and race of the inhabitants. It also includes data on income and occupation, as well as on general housing conditions.

Several different methods are used to estimate the

population of a community between the census-taking years. The arithmetic method and the geometric method are described below.

Arithmetic Method. By this method the average annual increase between the last two censuses is taken and used to compute the current population. For example, estimate the population of City A as of July 1, 1975. The 1960 census gave it a population of 100,000, and the 1970 census showed a population of 130,000, indicating an average annual increase of 3,000. Therefore, the estimated population as of July 1, 1975, would be:

Population as of July 1, 1970   130,000
Increase 1970-1975 = 3,000 × 5 =   15,000
Population as of July 1, 1975   145,000

It is obvious that this method (and, for that matter, most other methods) is open to inaccuracies, depending upon factors such as migration.

Geometric Method. This method assumes that the population increases according to the average *rate* of increase for the 10 intercensal years, as opposed to the average *number* used in the arithmetic method. Other methods in common use attempt to take the migration factor into consideration. As a rule, however, accurate information is difficult to secure.

Registration. A system of registration provides for the recording of births, deaths, marriages and, to a more limited extent, diseases. Birth and death records are important for a variety of reasons. For example, birth certificates are required when entering school, for obtaining various licenses, for social security benefits, voting, acquiring citizenship, entering military service, obtaining a passport and for insurance purposes.

Death certificates, on the other hand, are needed for claiming life insurance benefits and pensions. In addition, public, and for that matter private, agencies make extensive use of data, accumulated in and tabulated from these records, since these data form the basis for the computation of various mortality and morbidity rates. The tabulations also assist agencies to plan health programs, to evaluate the efficacy of existing programs and to compare the health status of one segment of the population or geographic area with another.

DISTRICT OF COLUMBIA DEPARTMENT OF PUBLIC HEALTH
CERTIFICATE OF LIVE BIRTH

BIRTH NO.

1. PLACE OF BIRTH					
Washington, D. C.	Name of Hospital or Institution (If not in Hospital, give street address)				

2. USUAL RESIDENCE OF MOTHER (Where does mother live?)

a. State	b. County		c. City, Town, or Location		
d. Street Address			e. Is Residence Inside City Limits? Yes ☐ No ☐		f. Is Residence on a Farm? Yes ☐ No ☐

CHILD

3. CHILD'S NAME (Type or Print)	(First)		(Middle)		(Last)
4. SEX Male ☐ Female ☐	5a. THIS BIRTH Single ☐ Twin ☐ Triplet ☐	5b. IF TWIN OR TRIPLET (This child born) 1st ☐ 2nd ☐ 3rd ☐		6. DATE OF BIRTH	(Month) (Day) (Year)

FATHER OF CHILD

7. NAME	(First)	(Middle)	(Last)	8. COLOR OR RACE
9. AGE (At time of this birth) YEARS	10. BIRTHPLACE (State or foreign country)	11a. USUAL OCCUPATION	11b. KIND OF BUSINESS OR INDUSTRY	

MOTHER OF CHILD

12. MAIDEN NAME	(First)	(Middle)	(Last)	13. COLOR OR RACE
14. AGE (At time of this birth) YEARS	15. BIRTHPLACE (State or foreign country)	16. CHILDREN PREVIOUSLY BORN TO THIS MOTHER (Do NOT include this child)		
17. INFORMANT (Full name) Parent ☐ Other ☐		a. How many OTHER children are now living?	b. How many OTHER children were born alive but are now dead?	c. How many children were stillborn (born dead after 20 weeks pregnancy)?

	I hereby certify that this child was born alive on the date stated above at the hour of _____M
NAME	18. SIGNATURE M. D.
ADDRESS	19. ADDRESS
CITY P. O. Zone STATE	20. DATE SIGNED

Fig. 1. *A*, Certificate of live birth employed in the District of Columbia.

SUPPLEMENTAL SECTION

BIRTH No.

(This portion of the certificate will be detached, filed apart, and used for statistical purposes only)

21. LEGITIMATE Yes ☐ No ☐	22. WEIGHT AT BIRTH _____ lbs. _____ ozs.	23. UNUSUAL NEED FOR RESUSCITATION Yes ☐ No ☐	24. CYANOSIS PERSISTING AFTER ONSET OF NORMAL RESPIRATION Yes ☐ No ☐
25a. ERYTHROBLASTOSIS Yes ☐ No ☐	25b. BIRTH INJURY Yes ☐ No ☐ (If yes, Describe) _____		
26. CONGENITAL MALFORMATIONS Yes ☐ No ☐ (If Yes, Describe) _____		27. OTHER CONDITIONS IN THE INFANT Yes ☐ No ☐ (If Yes, Describe) _____	

ITEMS RELATED TO PREGNANCY, LABOR, AND DELIVERY

28. FIRST DAY OF LAST MENSTRUAL PERIOD Date _____	29. PRENATAL CARE Yes ☐ No ☐ Date of First Visit _____ Approximate Number of Visits _____	30. ATTENDANT AT DELIVERY Private M. D. ☐ Resident Staff ☐ Other ☐

31. CONDITIONS OF PREGNANCY (Check Each Column)		32a. ONSET OF LABOR	32c. COMPLICATIONS OF LABOR
a. Directly Related	**b. Indirectly Related**	None ☐ Spontaneous ☐ Induced: Rupture of Membranes ☐ Oxytocic Drug ☐ Other (Specify) _____ ☐	None ☐ Placenta: Previa ☐ Abruptio ☐ Premature Separation ☐ Cord: Prolapse ☐ Anomaly ☐ Malpresentation: Breech ☐ Other ☐
None ☐ Preeclampsia ☐ Eclampsia ☐ Hypertension ☐ Nephritis ☐ Hemorrhage ☐ Premature Rupture of Membranes ☐ Other (Specify) _____ ☐	None ☐ Heart Disease ☐ Tuberculosis ☐ Diabetes ☐ Pyelitis ☐ Anemia (Hb under 10 gms) ☐ Virus Infection ☐ Other (Specify) _____ ☐	**32b. DURATION OF LABOR** None ☐ 1st and 2nd stage _____ hrs. 3rd stage _____ min.	Other Dystocia: Anomaly of the bony pelvis ☐ Fetal disproportion ☐ Uterine inertia ☐ Other Complication (Specify) _____ ☐

33. METHOD OF DELIVERY (Check One Only)				34. PLACENTA
Spontaneous ☐ Forceps: Low ☐ Rotation ☐ Mid ☐ High ☐	Cesarean Section Classical ☐ Low Cervical ☐ Extraperitoneal ☐ Hysterectomy ☐	Breech Extraction ☐ Version and Extraction ☐ Other (Specify) _____ ☐		Spontaneous expression ☐ Manual removal ☐ Abnormal placenta Yes ☐ No ☐

Fig. 1. *B,* Supplemental section to the certificate of live birth shown in Figure 1A. This section is used for statistical purposes only.

As a rule, reports of births and deaths must be made by a physician or by an undertaker respectively to a local registrar. The registrar has the responsibility of checking all certificates for completeness and accuracy and of mailing them to the office of the state headquarters. The registrar may be the local health officer; the state office is commonly the State Health Department.

Other Sources of Health Statistics. Health data can be secured from many other sources; in general, however, the material is not so reliable as that obtained from the aforementioned sources. Many diseases are reportable, although they provide a notoriously inadequate source of morbidity data. Health statistics are available from insurance companies, from hospital and clinic admissions, from schools and industry and from surveys, either local, specific, fact-finding surveys or

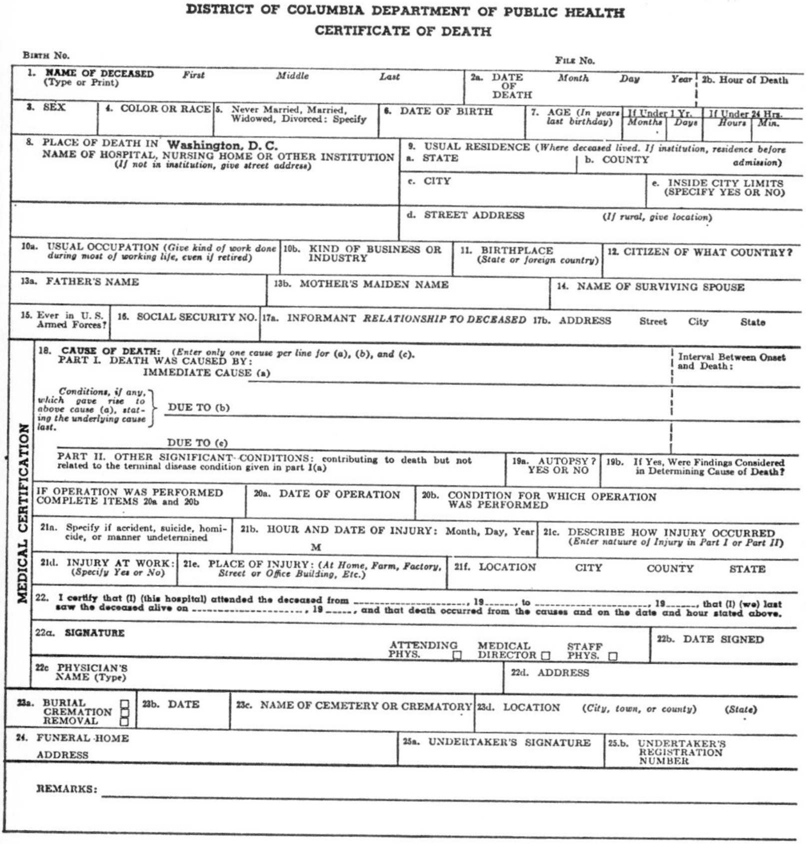

DISTRICT OF COLUMBIA DEPARTMENT OF PUBLIC HEALTH
CERTIFICATE OF DEATH

BIRTH No. FILE No.

1. NAME OF DECEASED (Type or Print) *First* *Middle* *Last*
2a. DATE OF DEATH *Month* *Day* *Year*
2b. Hour of Death
3. SEX
4. COLOR OR RACE
5. Never Married, Married, Widowed, Divorced: Specify
6. DATE OF BIRTH
7. AGE (*In years last birthday*) If Under 1 Yr. *Months* *Days* If Under 24 Hrs. *Hours* *Min.*
8. PLACE OF DEATH IN Washington, D. C. NAME OF HOSPITAL, NURSING HOME OR OTHER INSTITUTION (*If not in institution, give street address*)
9. USUAL RESIDENCE (*Where deceased lived. If institution, residence before admission*)
a. STATE
b. COUNTY
c. CITY
e. INSIDE CITY LIMITS (SPECIFY YES OR NO)
d. STREET ADDRESS (*If rural, give location*)
10a. USUAL OCCUPATION (*Give kind of work done during most of working life, even if retired*)
10b. KIND OF BUSINESS OR INDUSTRY
11. BIRTHPLACE (*State or foreign country*)
12. CITIZEN OF WHAT COUNTRY?
13a. FATHER'S NAME
13b. MOTHER'S MAIDEN NAME
14. NAME OF SURVIVING SPOUSE
15. Ever in U. S. Armed Forces?
16. SOCIAL SECURITY NO.
17a. INFORMANT *RELATIONSHIP TO DECEASED*
17b. ADDRESS Street City State

MEDICAL CERTIFICATION

18. CAUSE OF DEATH: (*Enter only one cause per line for (a), (b), and (c).*)
PART I. DEATH WAS CAUSED BY:
IMMEDIATE CAUSE (a)
Interval Between Onset and Death:
Conditions, if any, which gave rise to above cause (a), stating the underlying cause last.
DUE TO (b)
DUE TO (c)
PART II. OTHER SIGNIFICANT CONDITIONS: contributing to death but not related to the terminal disease condition given in part I(a)
19a. AUTOPSY? YES OR NO
19b. If Yes, Were Findings Considered in Determining Cause of Death?
IF OPERATION WAS PERFORMED COMPLETE ITEMS 20a and 20b
20a. DATE OF OPERATION
20b. CONDITION FOR WHICH OPERATION WAS PERFORMED
21a. Specify if accident, suicide, homicide, or manner undetermined
21b. HOUR AND DATE OF INJURY: Month, Day, Year M
21c. DESCRIBE HOW INJURY OCCURRED (*Enter natuure of Injury in Part I or Part II*)
21d. INJURY AT WORK: (*Specify Yes or No*)
21e. PLACE OF INJURY: (*At Home, Farm, Factory, Street or Office Building, Etc.*)
21f. LOCATION CITY COUNTY STATE
22. I certify that (I) (this hospital) attended the deceased from ____________, 19_____, to ____________, 19_____, that (I) (we) last saw the deceased alive on ____________, 19_____, and that death occurred from the causes and on the date and hour stated above.
22a. SIGNATURE ATTENDING PHYS. ☐ MEDICAL DIRECTOR ☐ STAFF PHYS. ☐
22b. DATE SIGNED
22c PHYSICIAN'S NAME (Type)
22d. ADDRESS
23a. BURIAL ☐ CREMATION ☐ REMOVAL ☐
23b. DATE
23c. NAME OF CEMETERY OR CREMATORY
23d. LOCATION (*City, town, or county*) (*State*)
24. FUNERAL HOME ADDRESS
25a. UNDERTAKER'S SIGNATURE
25.b. UNDERTAKER'S REGISTRATION NUMBER
REMARKS:

Fig. 2. Certificate of death employed in the District of Columbia.

national surveys. Many of these sources of data are, in fact, used in carrying out community health studies.

Reporting of Statistical Data

In order for statistics to be reported in a meaningful way, they must first be collected, then tabulated and correlated by machine. The information then available must be presented clearly and should be accompanied by appropriate written explanations. Aside from the common use of *tables* in presenting statistical data, the most usual form is graphic representation.

In a *line graph,* two variables are plotted as a series of points, and a line is drawn connecting them. A patient's temperature chart is a good example of a line graph. This type of chart is also used commonly to develop seasonal charts of individual diseases on the ba-

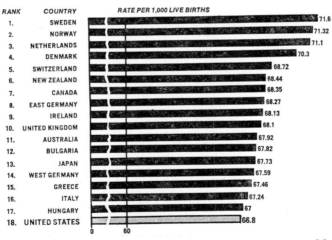

RANK	COUNTRY	RATE PER 1,000 LIVE BIRTHS
1.	SWEDEN	71.6
2.	NORWAY	71.32
3.	NETHERLANDS	71.1
4.	DENMARK	70.3
5.	SWITZERLAND	68.72
6.	NEW ZEALAND	68.44
7.	CANADA	68.35
8.	EAST GERMANY	68.27
9.	IRELAND	68.13
10.	UNITED KINGDOM	68.1
11.	AUSTRALIA	67.92
12.	BULGARIA	67.82
13.	JAPAN	67.73
14.	WEST GERMANY	67.59
15.	GREECE	67.46
16.	ITALY	67.24
17.	HUNGARY	67
18.	UNITED STATES	66.8

Fig. 3. The United States ranks 18th in the world in male life expectancy at birth. (Towards a Comprehensive Health Policy for the 1970's, HEW, May, 1971)

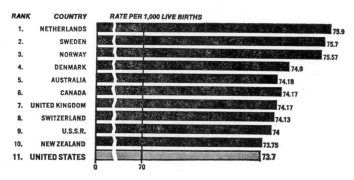

Fig. 4. The United States ranks 11th in female life expectancy at birth. (Towards a Comprehensive Health Policy for the 1970's, HEW, May, 1971)

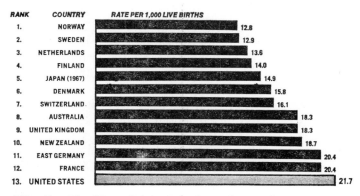

Fig. 5. The United States ranks 13th in infant mortality. (Towards a Comprehensive Health Policy for the 1970's, HEW, May, 1971)

sis of the number of cases occurring each week or month. These charts clearly show the trend of the disease, up or down, over a period of months or years. Similarly, annual deaths from, say, cancer of the cervix can be plotted with the trend observed over several years.

A *histogram* is similar to a line graph except that the points are replaced by perpendicular rectangles.

A *bar diagram* is similar to a histogram except that the thickness of the bars is of no consequence. It may be used, for example, to compare death rates from one particular disease in several different cities over a designated period of time.

Another useful form of presenting data is by means of maps, which are particularly valuable in demonstrating geographic distribution of a disease.

Rates Used in Statistical Studies

Some of the rates in common use are defined as follows:

1. Birth rates. The *crude birth rate* is the number of live births in a calendar year per 1,000 population (estimated as of the middle of that year).

The *age specific birth rate* is the number of live births to women in a selected age group per 1,000 women in that same age group.

2. Death rates. The *crude death rate* is the number of deaths reported in a calendar year per 1,000 population (estimated as of the middle of that year).

The *age specific death rate* is the number of deaths reported in a selected age group per 1,000 population in that same age group.

A *cause specific death rate* is the number of deaths from a specific cause in a calendar year per 100,000 population (estimated as of the middle of that year.)

Death rates, according to race, sex, and age: United States, 1976
(Data are based on the national vital registration system)

Age	All races			White			All other Total			All other Black		
	Both sexes	Male	Female	Both sexes	Male	Female	Both sexes	Male	Female	Both sexes	Male	Female
	Number of deaths per 100,000 resident population											
All ages[1]	889.6	1,007.0	778.3	899.4	1,010.4	793.6	824.8	983.5	680.0	886.2	1,051.8	735.7
Under 1 year	1,595.0	1,762.6	1,419.0	1,356.2	1,511.8	1,192.1	2,781.5	3,012.4	2,542.2	3,014.2	3,282.8	2,738.1
1–4 years	69.9	78.2	61.3	64.1	71.9	55.9	96.9	107.5	86.1	102.5	112.9	92.1
5–9 years	34.8	41.0	28.3	32.7	38.3	26.9	45.1	54.8	35.4	47.0	57.0	37.0
10–14 years	34.6	44.0	25.0	33.7	42.8	24.2	39.5	49.9	29.0	39.9	50.7	29.0
15–19 years	97.1	139.9	53.2	96.0	138.1	52.6	103.3	149.8	56.9	102.2	147.3	57.3
20–24 years	131.3	198.4	64.4	120.0	182.4	57.0	199.5	300.1	107.2	208.8	316.7	110.7
25–29 years	129.3	187.2	72.4	110.9	159.8	61.8	254.8	389.9	139.3	276.3	422.3	150.5
30–34 years	144.8	196.5	94.5	122.4	164.2	80.9	297.8	436.6	180.7	328.6	486.5	196.3
35–39 years	198.4	261.6	138.6	168.4	219.2	119.2	405.0	580.5	261.8	435.8	629.0	278.0
40–44 years	313.4	406.0	225.3	271.9	352.2	194.0	601.1	811.3	426.1	650.7	883.9	456.9
45–49 years	498.1	647.8	356.3	450.0	586.6	319.0	863.6	1,138.3	625.6	945.4	1,240.1	687.6
50–54 years	767.7	1,017.3	536.8	706.8	940.9	488.4	1,280.3	1,683.3	928.6	1,389.1	1,828.0	1,009.0
55–59 years	1,175.0	1,578.0	807.2	1,107.7	1,496.4	751.0	1,796.6	2,352.8	1,312.6	1,917.7	2,522.4	1,396.0
60–64 years	1,822.8	2,496.3	1,230.5	1,743.6	2,407.9	1,157.7	2,579.2	3,371.4	1,917.0	2,710.7	3,569.3	2,005.7
65–69 years	2,541.5	3,586.9	1,712.8	2,488.7	3,542.9	1,651.5	2,990.0	3,963.4	2,229.2	3,072.7	4,118.2	2,281.3
70–74 years	3,948.3	5,433.7	2,856.4	3,824.1	5,340.8	2,721.9	5,335.2	6,394.1	4,452.1	5,750.6	6,932.8	4,803.8
75–79 years	6,186.7	8,263.3	4,850.6	6,102.6	8,246.8	4,745.3	7,131.4	8,428.5	6,132.6	7,916.8	9,426.9	6,800.8
80–84 years	9,034.4	11,521.1	7,632.5	9,183.4	11,774.4	7,743.4	7,394.7	9,010.0	6,333.6	7,812.5	9,555.1	6,698.4
85 years and over	15,486.9	17,983.9	14,312.1	16,068.5	18,767.6	14,823.3	10,018.5	11,519.1	9,175.2	10,511.5	12,375.0	9,554.1

[1]Includes unknown age.

NOTE: Excludes deaths of nonresidents of the United States.

SOURCE: National Center for Health Statistics: *Vital Statistics of the United States, 1976*, Vol. II, Part A. Washington, U.S. Government Printing Office, Public Health Service, DHEW, Hyattsville, Md. Data computed by the Division of Analysis from data compiled by the Division of Vital Statistics.

Fig. 6. Vital statistics of the United States.

Infant mortality rate is the number of deaths of infants under one year of age during a calendar year per 1,000 live births during that year.

Maternal mortality rate is the number of deaths attributed to puerperal causes per 1,000 (or 10,000) live births.

Neonatal mortality rate is the number of deaths of infants under one month of age per 1,000 live births.

Perinatal mortality rate is the number of still births plus neonatal deaths during a calendar year per 1,000 total births occurring during that year.

Case fatality rate is the number of deaths from a specific cause per 100 (or 1,000) reported cases of the same condition.

3. *Morbidity rates.* The *incidence rate* is the number of reported cases of a given disease during a calendar year per 100,000 population (estimated as of the middle of that year).

Prevalence rate is the number of cases of a given illness at a particular time per 100,000 population at that same time.

Adjusted or standardized rates are often used in vital statistics. These are rates employed to compare two population groups in which the age distribution differs. Obviously, a high crude death rate in a population having a high percentage of persons over 65 years of age cannot be properly compared with the death rate in a population where the preponderance of persons is in the lower age groups. To compare these two populations, therefore, the age specific rates for each population are applied to a selected standard population. In this way, the number of deaths that would occur in each population if the age distributions were similar is obtained. The expected number of deaths in each population divided by the total number in the standard population will give comparable rates.

Some Statistical Terms

Frequency distribution is a statistical table which shows the number of observations in each classification group; for example, the number of deaths occurring in each age group.

The *mean* is the sum total of values of a series of observations divided by the number of observations.

The *median* is the center value in a series of observations ranging in order from high to low. There are as many values above the median as there are below it.

The *mode* is the value which occurs most frequently in a series of observations.

The *range* is the distance between the highest and lowest values in a series.

Average deviation is the mean of all the differences between each observation in a series and the median of the series.

Standard deviation is the most commonly used measurement of dispersion. In other words, it gives an indication as to whether or not all of the points center around the average or whether they are widespread. It is calculated by taking the squared deviations from the mean, dividing this sum by the number of items, and then taking the square root of the resulting quantity.

Illustration. Take, for example, an outbreak of food poisoning in which one is endeavoring to establish the incubation period. Assuming that one is presented with data indicating that 9 persons were involved and that the time interval from consumption of the meal to the time of onset of symptoms (in hours) is:

$$4 \quad 6 \quad 7 \quad 8 \quad 9 \quad 10 \quad 12 \quad 14 \quad 15$$

The *mean* is the sum of these numbers divided by 9 = approximately 9.5. The *median* is 9. The *average deviation* is 9 (the median) less each of the above numbers; these are then added and divided by 8 (the total number of values, less the median) = 3.25. The *standard deviation* is 3.7.

Interpreting Statistical Data

It is important to recognize and appreciate the fact that in any scientific study, when a series of observations are made, inevitable differences and inconsistencies will be found. This is usually called *variability*. It may be due to many factors, such as sampling variations or experimental error; but irrespective of the reason, it is important to recognize that one is dealing not in certainties but in probabilities.

A scientific study should be carried out by a carefully and systematically developed procedure. In analyzing the data presented as being evidence supporting or not supporting a particualr hypothesis, one must critically evaluate the information with the following questions in mind:

1. Could the results be accounted for by normal differences that may well occur in samples taken from the same population base?
2. Are the results due to bias, for example, in the methods used to acquire the data? For example, if a questionnaire was used, were the questions of the type that might tend to bias?
3. Are the results due to inappropriate comparisons? For example, comparing data from hospitalized patients with those not hospitalized may be quite improper, just as it is inaccurate to compare crude death rates of two population groups without

knowing the age distribution of the groups' members.

4. Is the method of selecting cases equitable? It is essential that any comparisons being made between two groups must be based on groups with essentially similar characteristics.

5. Are the results due to factors which have not thus far been substantiated?

6. Are the results due to factors already known, such as age and sex? For example, lung cancer is already known to be much more common in men than in women; therefore, differences in incidence are to be expected for this reason alone.

Another important factor in analyzing data concerns the question of whether or not there is an adequate control group; this factor is often missing in some of the published material. It is not always easy to acquire a statistically valid control group, since the control must be essentially identical with the study group; this is often difficult to achieve, particularly in experiments involving human beings.

Tests of Statistical Significance

In examining published data purporting to show certain results, it is essential for the student to ask himself the question, "Can the results demonstrated be attributed to chance variation?" Tests of statistical significance have as their objective the determination of whether or not the observation is sufficiently different from what would normally be expected to probably be due to something other than chance. Several tests are in common use, but the one which will be described here is known as the *Chi square test* (x^2).

The following tables, adapted from Hilleboe and Larimore's *Preventive Medicine*, will illustrate its use:

Mortality under 28 Days among Premature Births in Three Different Hospitals

Hospital	Total	Died Under 28 Days	Survived 28 Days or More	Death Rate Under 28 Days Per 1,000 Premature Births
A	622	124	498	199
B	831	182	649	219
C	499	137	362	275
Total	1,952	443	1,509	227

A Chi square test can be used to answer the question, "Are death rates under 28 days among prematures in the three hospitals different from what one would expect on the basis of sampling variation?"

One proceeds as follows:

1. Obtain the expected value for the under 28-day mortality rate by computing the rate for all three hospitals combined by dividing total deaths under 28 days by total premature births:

   Expected death rate under 28 days $= 443/1,952$
   $= 227/1,000$

2. Obtain the expected survival rate by subtracting the death rate from 1,000:

   Expected survival rate $= 1,000 - 227 = 773/1,000$

3. For each hospital, obtain the expected number of deaths and survivors by multiplying the total premature births in each hospital by the expected under 28-day death rate ($227/1,000$) and by the expected survival rate ($773/1,000$), respectively. The results are shown below:

Expected Mortality under 28 Days among Premature Births in Three Different Hospitals

Hospital	Total	Died under 28 Days (Expected)	Survived 28 Days or More (Expected)
A	622	(a) 141	(d) 481
B	831	(b) 189	(e) 642
C	499	(c) 113	(f) 386
Totals	1,952	442	1,509

4. For each cell (a) through (f) obtain the difference between the actual number of events and the expected number of events. For example:

cell (a) 124 − 141 = 17
cell (b) 182 − 189 =   7
cell (c) 137 − 113 = 24
and so on through cells (d) thru (f)

5. Square each difference. For example:

cell (a) = $(17)^2$ = 289
and so on through cells (b) thru (f)

6. Divide each square difference by the number in the corresponding cell in the *expected* table. For example:

cell (a) 289/141 = 2.05
cell (b)   49/189 = 0.26
and so on through cells (c) thru (f)

7. Add the values obtained for all 6 cells. In this example this adds up to 9.58.
8. To determine the significance of this value consult a table of Chi square probability. It will be found that the calculated value of Chi square = 9.58 and

lies between the 0.01 and the 0.001 probability levels.

9. The difference in rates among these three hospitals would, therefore, occur less than one time in a hundred if the only factor affecting these differences was chance. On this basis, one would assume that the differences were due to some influence other than chance.

REFERENCES

Confrey, E. A.: *Administration of Community Health Services,* International City Managers Association, 1963.

Hill, A. Bradford: *Principles of Medical Statistics,* 9th Ed., New York, Oxford University Press, 1971.

Kinch, S., & Amos, F. B.: Vital Statistics, in *Preventive Medicine,* Hilleboe and Larimore, 2nd Ed., Philadelphia, W. B. Saunders Co., 1965.

Physicians' Handbook on Medical Certification: Death, Fetal Death, Birth. National Center for Health Statistics. U.S. Dept. of HEW, 1968.

Swaroop, S.: *Introduction to Health Statistics,* Edinburgh, E. & S. Livingstone, Ltd., 1960.

Chapter 3

Principles in the Prevention of Communicable Disease

Extent of the Problem

Both morbidity and mortality from communicable diseases have fallen drastically in the past half century. In 1900, approximately a third of all deaths in the United States resulted from communicable diseases. Today, less than 1 in 10 deaths is attributable to this cause. In spite of this great decline, communicable diseases continue to be an important cause of illness and death in this country and, even more so, in many other countries of the world. In fact, life expectancy in some other less developed countries is, perhaps, half of what it is in the United States; in those countries, diseases such as malaria and schistosomiasis are common and take a considerable toll of human life. Diseases such as cholera are still endemic in certain parts of the world, *e.g.*, India, while typhoid fever and the dysenteries are very common in many countries, such as Mexico and Japan. Yaws is extremely common in the tropics; even smallpox, plague and yellow fever still occur. It is of interest that the leading cause of death in the world today is not heart disease, but malaria.

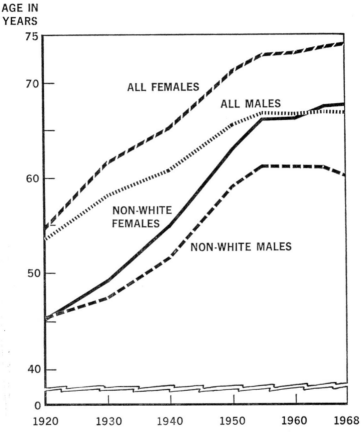

Fig. 7. Expectation of life at birth, 1920-1968. (Towards a Comprehensive Health Policy for the 1970's, HEW, May, 1971)

In this country, certainly, serious communicable diseases have practically been eradicated, but diseases such as tuberculosis and syphilis are still common. Many other less serious but potentially disabling illnesses (because of the possible complications which may result) still occur widely; examples of these are colds, measles and streptococcal sore throat. In addition, outbreaks of other diseases occur with some frequency; these include encephalitis and hepatitis.

Aside from the sickness and death produced by these and other communicable diseases, enormous economic losses result from sickness-absenteeism from work.

Infection and Resistance

Infection occurs as a result of penetration of the tissues by pathogenic organisms or particles. Soon after infection has taken place, antibodies are produced. The result of this battle between infectious forces and the body defenses may be death of the host, a period of sickness followed by recovery, existence of infection without any apparent sickness or a latent infection better known as the carrier state.

While the existence of sickness in a person may be obvious, undiagnosed illnesses and carriers of disease are of great importance in epidemiology because the number of these may exceed that of persons in whom sickness is obvious. It is often through the medium of the unrecognized cases and the carriers that the disease spreads. This is one of the mean reasons that isolation and quarantine, once practiced extensively and thought to be among the most important means of preventing the spread of disease, now are not usually considered of great value. The other important contributing factor to the spread of disease is the incubation period. Here, again, is an interval during which the disease is present but unrecognized while, nevertheless, the individual may be able to spread his inapparent infection to others.

The essential requirements for establishment of a parasitic relationship between the host and the infectious agent are:

1. An agent
2. A reservoir
3. A susceptible host
4. A vehicle for transmission

The agent includes many varieties of bacteria, rickettsia, viruses, worms and fungi. Not all agents are pathogenic to man; some, in fact, are useful rather than dangerous.

A reservoir may be a human being or an animal. Arthropods often serve as reservoirs, as do plants or other matter in which the agent can live and grow.

A susceptible host is one who does not possess sufficient resistance to a particular pathogen. Susceptibility is dependent upon many factors, including the host's previous contact experience with a particular agent, his natural or acquired immunity against it and his current state of health. For example, the existence of an already debilitating disease may render the host's powers of resistance relatively ineffective. The agent must also be able to find a portal of entry into and exit from the host. The portal of entrance is usually the same as that of exit.

The vehicles for transmission constitute the mechanism by which the agent is carried from the reservoir to the susceptible host. These are air, milk, water or food, and insects.

Spread of Infectious Diseases

It is necessary now to consider in detail the three *major* factors involved in the spread of infectious diseases, namely, the agent, the host, and the environment.

The Agent. Of importance are the agent's characteristics, including factors such as its viability and resistance, motility, nutritional and reproductive requirements. These characteristics vary greatly; for example, some bacteria produce spores which can survive under normally adverse conditions for long periods. Extremes of temperature are usually harmful to bacteria, while viruses tend to die at room temperature.

The manner in which the agent invades, gains entrance and lives within the host varies with the agent; for example, the *Entamoeba histolytica* gains entrance by ingestion, while the arthropods usually damage the host's skin by biting.

The pathogenicity of agents also varies greatly, some producing a much more virulent reaction than others. Fungi, for example, are usually only moderately pathogenic, while the virus of rabies is extremely high in its pathogenicity.

The ability of the agent to stimulate the host to produce antibodies (antigenicity) is also subject to much variation. Bacteria are generally antigenic, while the rickettsiae usually produce life-long immunity.

Transmission of disease to the host may be effected by several means:

1. *From person to person.* For disease to spread in this way, some kind of contact between people is required. This may be direct contact; for example, the disease may be spread via the respiratory tract as a result of inhalation of infected droplets suspended in the

air. On the other hand, contact may be indirect, an example being afforded by the spread of gastrointestinal diseases through the medium of flies.

2. *From a common vehicle.* In this mechanism, disease is spread through such vehicles as water, milk or food in which the agent usually is able to thrive. This is the common mode of spread of gastrointestinal infections. Outbreaks of disease resulting from spread by common vehicles are generally explosive; in other words, the outbreak occurs suddenly and affects a considerable number of persons over a relatively short time span.

3. *Through vectors.* Many diseases are spread through the medium of an arthropod vector. Often, however, the vector is dependent upon an animal reservoir. For example, typhus fever is a disease of rats, transmitted to man via the rat flea or the louse.

The Host. Many characteristics of the host have an impact upon the development of infectious disease.

1. *Age.* Babies are often immune to some diseases because of antibodies acquired from their mothers. Other diseases appear to be particularly dangerous in young children, for example, pertussis and measles.

2. *Heredity.* Many individuals appear to have some degree of inherited immunity to infectious disease. On the other hand, certain races appear to be particularly susceptible to tuberculosis. Sometimes this may be confused with the well-known principle that when a communicable disease has been absent from an area for some considerable time, the number of susceptible individuals increases, so that if the organism is subsequently introduced into that area a large number of cases occur. An example is afforded by the measles epidemic which swept through Greenland in 1951.

3. *Habits and Customs.* Clearly, these are important

factors in the dissemination of communicable disease. For example, the means by which a family or community disposes of its human waste may be the means by which enteric disease occurs and spreads. Similarly, people in areas where unpasteurized milk is consumed are likely to be the victims of several different diseases spread through the medium of this milk. By the same token, promiscuity may lead to the development of venereal disease; also, certain occupations or activities will expose the persons engaged in them to diseases such as anthrax.

4. *Immunity*. The host has several ways of protecting himself against the agent of infectious disease. Aside from those protective devices inherently possessed by everyone, such as the skin, the cilia, the liver, the lungs, and the spleen, each individual has a defense mechanism brought about by interaction between the infectious agent and the antibodies produced by the host. This is called immunity.

Active immunity occurs when the body develops its own antibodies in response to a specific antigen (agent). It may be naturally acquired as a result of direct infection, or it may be artificially acquired as a result of immunization (purposeful injection of an antigen to stimulate the production of antibodies).

In passive immunity, the body either acquires antibodies in ready-made form, as do babies from their mothers, or artificially by direct injection, usually in the form of gamma globulin.

Active immunity takes time to develop but is of much longer duration than passive immunity.

The Environment. Clearly, different environments contribute variously to disease; for example, malaria-producing mosquitoes live in low, swampy areas, whereas desert regions may be more suitable for fungi or bacterial spores. Similarly, the biologic environment is of great importance. Many animals develop diseases that can be transmitted to man. Certain birds transmit psittacosis, fish may be infected with worms, while the soil may contain the spores of tetanus and histoplasma.

The Action between Agent and Host. After the agent gains the portal of entry to the host, it may lodge and multiply but produce no immediate, obvious reaction; an example of this is seen in primary syphilis, where the chancre takes some three weeks to develop following entry of the spirochete. On the other hand, the agent may lodge, multiply and produce evident signs of disease. The body defense mechanisms come into play, and a battle ensues in which the outcome may be elimination of the agent with recovery of the host, death of the host, or evident recovery although the agent is retained in the body of the host (carrier state).

When the agent first gains entry, there is an incubation period before obvious signs of illness appear in the host. During this time, the agent is multiplying and perhaps producing its toxins, while the host is mobilizing his defenses. This defense mechanism may be sufficiently powerful to produce a subclinical case in which no infection can be recognized. Much depends upon the dose of the infectious agent. Large doses are particularly likely to produce a more severe reaction.

Prevention of Communicable Diseases

Preventive techniques may be directed to the source case, to the environment or to the host.

The Source Case. The chief method of control of the source case involves the isolation of the host to prevent him from transmitting the infection to other susceptible persons. However, it is clear from what has already been stated that isolation of the source case is not a particularly effective method of preventing the spread of disease. This is because infectivity is present during part of the incubation period before symptoms are recognizable and because of the number of subclinical cases. A similar situation prevails when a considerable number of cases of an infectious disease occur in a school. The tendency on the part of school authorities is usually to close the school in order to avoid further dissemination of the disease. As a rule, however, this will not prevent the disease from spreading.

On the other hand, quarantine may be of some value and has been effectively practiced in diseases such as cholera. In this instance, the secondarily infected contacts are kept from other persons during the incubation period and before they become obviously sick.

The Environment. Great success has attended many of the preventive measures traditionally practiced in the environment. For example, pasteurization of milk has been extremely effective in preventing the spread of milk-borne ailments, while purification of water supplies and improvements in methods of sewage disposal have been effective in reducing the prevalence of enteric diseases. Control of arthropod vectors by methods such as drainage of swampy areas to eliminate breeding sites for mosquitoes, rat-proofing of buildings, the use of insecticides, screening and the use of insect repellants have all played an important role in preventing diseases such as malaria, typhus and yellow fever.

Proper food handling, adequate refrigeration and, in some cases, thorough cooking of the food also serve to reduce the extent of food-borne disease.

The Host. Steps taken to improve the general health status of the population and of individual persons are of importance in maintaining body defenses at a high level. In this connection, improvement of nutrition and personal hygiene, and the reduction of over-crowding and of excessive fatigue are important. A healthful emotional climate may also play a role in influencing the development and course of communicable disease.

Perhaps the most important specific protective measure of value in preventing infectious disease is immunization. Several diseases can be effectively prevented by prophylactic injection of toxoid or vaccine at intervals which vary with the disease. Temporary passive immunization, by which antibodies are injected through the medium of gamma globulin, is of limited value in preventing certain diseases. The short duration (5 to 6 weeks) of its effect renders this procedure useful primarily in isolated instances where there is an urgent need for immediate protection as, for example, in the case of a pregnant woman exposed to rubella.

Diseases in which immunization is of primary importance include smallpox, diphtheria, measles, pertussis, tetanus, poliomyelitis and rubella. The control of poliomyelitis brought about by immunization programs is excellent testimony to the value of this technique. In the United States, the annual number of cases reported averaged close to 39,000 from 1950 to 1954, before polio vaccination programs became general. Only 20 cases were reported in 1977.

There are many other diseases against which immunization is practiced. While this procedure may be useful in helping to prevent illness in some cases, it should not be thought that immunization is equally effective in all instances. Examples include influenza, typhoid, cholera, plague and tuberculosis.

Secondary prevention is of considerable importance in preventing complications in patients suffering from a communicable disease. This has been greatly simplified by use of the wide variety of antibiotics generally available. Antibiotics have played an important role in reducing mortality from secondary infections, particularly in measles and pertussis.

Role of the Health Department

Clearly, the official health department has an important part to play in controlling the spread of communicable diseases. Apart from the development of community-wide immunization programs, case-finding (as in tuberculosis by means of x-ray film surveys of high risk groups) and health department activities in environmental sanitation make important contributions. So, too, the health department is in a key position to follow up and arrange for examination of contacts of cases of tuberculosis and venereal disease, as well as to make epidemiologic investigations of disease outbreaks and to establish appropriate control measures. The health department laboratory, too, performs a valuable service by examining human secretions, blood and urine, and by checking samples of water, milk and food for evidence of contamination.

PREVENTION OF SPECIFIC DISEASES

No attempt is being made in this book to deal with the exact methods of prevention of specific diseases, since this is dealt with in textbooks of medicine and more comprehensive texts in the field of public health and preventive medicine. However, because of the high morbidity and particular significance attached to tuberculosis and venereal disease and in view of the extensive traditional involvement of public health agencies in their control, the prevention of these diseases will be discussed.

TUBERCULOSIS CASES BY REGION, 1976 AND 1977

Area	1976 Cases	1976 Case Rate	1977 Cases	1977 Case Rate
United States	32,105	15.0	30,145	13.9
New England				
Maine	72	6.7	82	7.6
New Hampshire	34	4.1	22	2.6
Vermont	36	7.6	37	7.7
Massachusetts	676	11.6	647	11.2
Rhode Island	82	8.8	78	8.3
Connecticut	227	7.3	247	7.9
Middle Atlantic				
New York	3,072	17.0	2,434	13.6
New Jersey	1,201	16.4	1,162	15.9
Pennsylvania	1,511	12.7	1,282	10.9
East North Central				
Ohio	926	8.7	845	7.9
Indiana	544	10.3	560	10.5
Illinois	1,711	15.2	1,727	15.4
Michigan	1,349	14.8	1,290	14.1
Wisconsin	225	4.9	181	3.9
West North Central				
Minnesota	213	5.4	211	5.3
Iowa	115	4.0	99	3.4
Missouri	568	11.9	497	10.4
North Dakota	40	6.2	32	4.9
South Dakota	62	9.0	58	8.4
Nebraska	58	3.7	42	2.7
Kansas	135	5.8	153	6.6
South Atlantic				
Delaware	82	14.1	67	11.5
Maryland	925	22.3	827	20.0
District of Columbia	319	45.4	342	49.6
Virginia	821	16.3	742	14.4
West Virginia	263	14.4	239	12.9
North Carolina	1,220	22.3	1,042	18.9
South Carolina	589	20.7	643	22.4
Georgia	824	16.6	916	18.1
Florida	1,630	19.4	1,674	19.8

TUBERCULOSIS CASES BY AGE AND RACE, 1976

Age	Total	White	Other
0-4	998	509	489
5-14	777	342	435
15-24	2,442	1,086	1,356
25-44	8,452	3,784	4,668
45-64	11,006	6,640	4,366
65+	8,430	6,088	2,342
Total	32,105	18,449	13,656

TUBERCULOSIS CASES BY SEX AND RACE, 1976

Sex	Total	White	Other
Male	20,933	12,219	8,714
Female	11,172	6,230	4,942
Total	32,105	18,449	13,656

Age	White Male	White Female	Other Male	Other Female
0-14	423	428	446	478
15-44	2,884	1,986	3,617	2,407
45-64	4,923	1,717	3,098	1,268
65+	3,989	2,099	1,553	789
Total	12,219	6,230	8,714	4,942

TUBERCULOSIS CASE RATES BY AGE, RACE, AND SEX, 1976

Age	Total	White Total	White Male	White Female	Other Total	Other Male	Other Female
All Ages	15.0	9.9	13.4	6.5	48.0	64.2	33.3
0-4	6.5	4.0	4.0	4.1	18.2	17.5	18.9
5-14	2.1	1.1	1.0	1.2	7.1	6.8	7.5
15-24	6.0	3.1	3.2	3.0	22.7	22.4	22.9
25-44	15.4	7.9	9.7	6.1	66.8	92.9	44.9
45-64	25.2	17.0	26.2	8.4	95.7	146.5	51.8
65+	36.8	29.2	47.2	17.0	111.3	171.4	65.8

East South Central

State				
Kentucky	586	17.1	719	20.8
Tennessee	902	21.4	864	20.1
Alabama	824	22.5	704	19.1
Mississippi	434	18.4	460	19.3
West South Central				
Arkansas	444	21.1	392	18.3
Louisiana	614	16.0	615	15.7
Oklahoma	399	14.4	305	10.9
Texas	2,454	19.7	2,326	18.1
Mountain				
Montana	51	6.8	68	8.9
Idaho	37	4.5	38	4.4
Wyoming	20	5.1	20	4.9
Colorado	174	6.7	149	5.7
New Mexico	181	15.5	152	12.8
Arizona	405	17.8	358	15.6
Utah	60	4.9	43	3.4
Nevada	42	6.9	58	9.2
Pacific				
Washington	378	10.5	384	10.5
Oregon	197	8.5	171	7.2
California	3,620	16.8	3,465	15.8
Alaska	88	23.0	92	22.6
Hawaii	665	75.0	584	65.3
Guam	46	46.0	67	67.0
Puerto Rico	398	12.8	—	—
Virgin Islands	6	6.1	7	7.1
Trust Territory of the Pacific Islands	63	49.4	77	60.3

SOURCE: Center for Disease Control: *Reported Morbidity and Mortality in the United States: Annual Summary 1977.* Vol. 26, No. 53. Sept. 1978

Fig. 8. Tuberculosis Cases and Cases per 100,000 Population by Geographic Division and by State, United States, 1976 and 1977; and by Age, Race, and Sex, United States, 1976

Tuberculosis

Even today, when morbidity and mortality from tuberculosis have greatly declined, this disease remains the most important communicable disease in the United States in terms of its ability to cause chronic disability and death. It occurs with great frequency in areas where the standard of living is low, and it is generally common among the underprivileged.

It is because of its importance as a prime cause of disability and death that tuberculosis has assumed singular importance in public health circles over a period of many years. Efforts by public health authorities to control the spread of this disease can be traced back to the beginning of this century with the establishment of the National Tuberculosis Association. Soon thereafter, official public health agencies became very active in taking steps aimed at case finding, isolation, treatment and other methods of controlling the spread of this disease.

Improvements in general nutrition, housing conditions and measures to raise the standard of living are important in reducing the prevalence of tuberculosis. More specific measures, however, are aimed predominantly at finding the unknown cases. This is accomplished by routine chest x-ray films particularly of those segments of the population known to have a high incidence of tuberculosis, such as jail inmates, and by tuberculin testing programs. One of the most important sources of new cases, however, arises from continued and careful surveillance of contacts of known cases of the disease.

Once diagnosis is suspected or established, thorough treatment of the patient is indicated. Until recently, hospitalization was considered preferable in the initial stages of treatment because:

1. It removes the patient from the immediate community, thereby reducing the possibility of his spreading the disease to others.
2. It ensures proper rest and treatment of the patient himself with a view towards speeding his recovery in a way not normally possible in a home environment.

However, with the advent and increasing use of antituberculosis drugs and the concomitant resistance of many patients to prolonged hospitalization, the modern tendency is to treat the tuberculous patient as an outpatient and to endeavor to maintain him under close surveillance and to render him noncommunicable as rapidly as possible through a combination of drug therapy and a reasonable living regimen. Continued medical supervision is essential, together with regular public health nursing service aimed primarily at ensuring that the patient is taking the necessary precautions to prevent spreading the disease to others and that he is taking the drugs as prescribed.

One other preventive measure should be mentioned. This involves the use of isoniazid prophylaxis, particularly in children with primary tuberculosis. More recently, isoniazid has been used among adults with positive reactions to tuberculin tests, mostly in areas where the incidence of tuberculosis is high. This prophylactic measure has given some indication that it is of real value in reducing the number of future cases of tuberculosis.

Finally, in spite of the controversy raging around the use of BCG vaccination against tuberculosis, there is little question that the procedure does, in fact, provide some protection against the disease. The main question revolves around the indications for the use of BCG vaccination. The prevailing opinion in the United States today is that it is not indicated at all in low-risk tuberculosis areas, but that it may well be of value in high-risk groups, such as household contacts. Clearly, its effect in producing a positive reaction to the tuberculin test, which therefore renders the use of this test of little value as a control measure, must be considered.

Venereal Disease

As with tuberculosis, public health interest in venereal disease control dates back many years. This is primarily due to the great social importance of venereal diseases, coupled with their high prevalence. From 1947 to 1957, reported cases of primary and secondary syphilis in the United States indicated a drastically downward trend. Since then, however, the number of cases of syphilis has increased rather sharply. The incidence of gonorrhea, too, has shown a dramatic increase in recent years. Many reasons have been cited although these are essentially conjectural; they include lowering of moral standards, an increase in homosexuality, and lack of funds available to assist in controlling the disease.

Control of the venereal diseases must include a search for the unknown cases. In this connection, contact investigation is most important and is one of the roles which the health department is usually best equipped to play. Every sex contact of a person having venereal disease must be located, examined and treated. This necessitates good case reporting by physicians. As a matter of fact, nowhere in the field of public health is a good relationship between private medical practitioners and the official health agency more important. A good case-finding program also requires blood-testing programs in patients admitted to hospitals and particularly in high incidence groups, such as jail inmates, followed by reporting of positive reactions to the health department. The recently introduced technique of cluster epidemiology investigates all the social contacts of the source case and has been quite effective. Adequate diagnostic and treatment facilities must be available; special facilities may be required to handle homosexuals. Health education programs geared to the public at large, but including school children, are an important ingredient of the venereal disease control program.

REFERENCES

Kane, R. L.: *The Challenges of Community Medicine,* New York, Springer Publishing Co., 1974.

Leavell, H. R., and Clark, E. G.: *Preventive Medicine for the Doctor in his Community,* 3rd Ed., New York, McGraw-Hill Book Co., 1958.

Raffel, S.: *Immunity,* 2nd Ed., New York, Appleton-Century-Crofts, Inc., 1961.

Top, F. H., and Wehrle, P. F.: *Communicable and Infectious Diseases,* 8th Ed., St. Louis, C. V. Mosby Co., 1976.

Chapter 4

Principles in the Prevention of Chronic Disease

Extent of the Problem

As a result, primarily, of the great decrease in deaths from communicable diseases, a decrease brought about by improved methods of diagnosis, better treatment, vastly higher standards of sanitation, nutrition and housing, and various preventive measures including immunization, there has been a radical change in the leading causes of death in this country. In 1900, the commonest causes of death were tuberculosis, pneumonia and influenza, diarrhea and enteritis. Today, these causes have been entirely supplanted by cardiovascular diseases and cancer. Longevity has increased markedly, and more and more persons are surviving to an old age. Today, approximately 11% of the population of the United States is aged 65 or over, as compared to about 4% in 1900. During this time, too, the population of the country has grown rapidly so that the absolute numbers of those 65 and over have increased greatly. By the year 2,000, it is expected that some 40% of the popu-

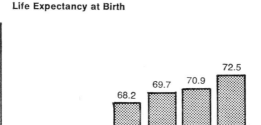

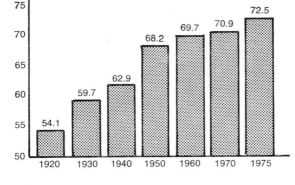

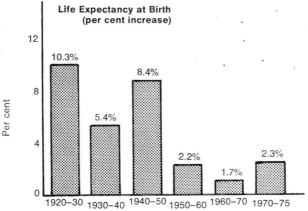

Source: U.S. National Center for Health Statistics, Vital Statistics of the U.S.

Fig. 9.   Life expectancy

lation of the United States will be 45 years of age or over.

As our citizens grow into middle and old age, they enter the period of life in which the chronic diseases become increasingly prevalent. These are the ages at which cardiovascular disease, cancer, arthritis and rheumatism, diabetes and glaucoma are most apt to occur.

The Commission on Chronic Illness has defined chronic illness as comprising "all impairments or deviations from normal which have one or more of the following characteristics: are permanent, leave residual disability, are caused by nonreversible pathological alterations, require special training of the patient for rehabilitation, may be expected to require a long period of supervision, observation or care."

Age	Year					
	1900	1920	1940	1960	1970	1977
	Population in thousands					
Total population—	76,094	106,461	132,122	179,979	203,810	216,332
	Per cent distribution					
<5 years	12.1	10.9	8.0	11.3	8.4	7.0
5–14 years	22.3	20.8	16.9	19.9	20.0	16.8
15–24 years	19.6	17.7	18.2	13.4	17.6	18.9
25–34 years	16.0	16.4	16.2	12.6	12.3	15.2
35–44 years	12.2	13.5	13.9	13.4	11.3	10.9
45–54 years	8.5	9.9	11.8	11.4	11.4	10.8
55–64 years	5.3	6.2	8.1	8.7	9.2	9.4
65 + years	4.1	4.6	6.8	9.3	9.9	10.9

NOTE: All years except for 1940 refer to the resident population.
SOURCE: Selected data from the Bureau of the Census

Fig. 10. Population distribution for selected years 1900-1977.

While exact figures concerning chronic disease morbidity are not easy to secure, interviews carried out by the National Health Survey have revealed that some 40% of the population of the United States have one or more chronic conditions. These studies have clearly demonstrated the increasing frequency of these diseases with advancing age. It has been estimated that there are close to 6 million persons in the United States with chronic disabilities sufficiently serious to require care. More than a third of these individuals are 65 years of age or older.

During the past 35 years or so the central cities have tended to lose population to the suburbs, while the Negro population of the city has substantially increased. Concurrent with these changes are the following facts: Mortality rates and incidence of reportable diseases are higher than for the suburban and rural sections of the country. Infant mortality rate is much higher while the tuberculosis and venereal disease rates are several times higher than for other sections of the country. Surprisingly to some, it will usually be found that death rates from cancer, heart disease and accidents are considerably above state and national levels. Illegitimacy rates are far greater and while comparable statistics are not available, there is no doubt that alcoholism, drug addiction, and mental illness morbidity are high.

Chronic illnesses have plagued man since the beginning of history. Until recent times, they were regarded as inescapable. Now, some forms of chronic disability have been reduced or even eliminated, for example, poliomyelitis, much of tuberculosis and chronic osteomyelitis. At the same time, the prevalence of chronic illness has increased primarily because many people who would have previously died from illnesses once thought fatal now survive into the years when chronic disease is most common. Eighty per cent of people 65 or older have at least one chronic condition and more than half of these are limited, to some extent, in their activities. Two million Americans have survived strokes with varying degrees of residual impairment; arthritis affects some 12 million persons; approximately 4½ million persons in the United States are known to have diabetes; more than a million have glaucoma.

There are several important factors which have some bearing on the chronic disease problem. In the first, as one goes down the socioeconomic ladder, mortality rates from most important chronic diseases tend to rise; this gradient is also reflected in morbidity figures. The National Health Survey has shown that chronic limitation of mobility has a much higher prevalence in those with low family income than in those whose income is much greater.

A second factor of importance is that of nutrition. Certainly, nutritional deficiency diseases are well known, but the question of obesity is one which has been engaging the increasing attention of research workers. Life insurance tables have shown that, in general, the greater the degree of overweight, the higher the death rate from cardiovascular disease and diabetes.

A third factor clearly shown to be of importance is that of cigarette smoking. Several studies have revealed higher mortality rates among cigarette smokers than among non-smokers, and the greater the amount of smoking the higher the mortality rate. While most attention has been given to the association between smoking and lung cancer, there is also mounting evidence of a relationship to both respiratory and cardiovascular disease.

Rank, 1976	Cause of death and category numbers of the Eighth Revision International Class-ification of Diseases, Adapted, 1965	Number of deaths, 1976	Rate per 100,000 population 1976	1900
	All causes	1,909,440	889.6	1,719.1
1	Diseases of heart 390–398,402,404,410–429	723,878	337.2	137.4
2	Malignant neoplasms, including neoplasms of lymphatic and hematopoietic tissues 140–209	377,312	175.8	64.0
3	Cerebrovascular diseases 430–438	188,623	87.9	106.9
4	Accidents E800–E949	100,761	46.9	72.3
5	Influenza and pneumonia 470–474,480–486	61,866	28.8	202.2
6	Diabetes mellitus 250	34,508	16.1	11.0
7	Cirrhosis of liver 571	31,453	14.7	12.5
8	Arteriosclerosis 440	29,366	13.7	—
9	Suicide E950–E959	26,832	12.5	10.2
10	Certain causes of mortality in early infancy[1] ..760,769.2,769.4–772,774–778	24,809	11.6	62.6

[1] Relates to birth injuries, asphyxia, infections of newborn, ill-defined diseases, immaturity, etc.

Source: National Center for Health Statistics: Selected data from Division of Vital Statistics.

Fig. 11. Deaths and death rates for the 10 leading causes of death in 1976 and death rates for these same causes in 1900.

Every year approximately 20,000 persons in the United States die from rheumatic fever and its compli-cations. Judicious use of antibiotics could undoubtedly prevent many of these deaths. The Papanicolaou smear has been known and available for several years; yet each year, many women die because cervical cancer was not detected at an early stage. The U.S. Public Health Service has estimated that in spite of simple tests readily available for the early detection of diabetes and glaucoma, some 4 million cases of diabetes and

3

well over a half a million cases of glaucoma currently remain undetected in this country.

It has been estimated that up to 50% of the morbidity seen in our long-term facilities and rehabilitation centers is due, not to the disease itself, but to the immobilization of all or part of the patient's body. The importance of early active physical therapy is obvious, particularly when dealing with older persons where lack of mobility can most readily produce early disability. The overall goal of rehabilitation is to restore the individual so that he may be able to resume useful employment and independent living. On the other hand, partial rehabilitative gains may be useful, even if only part of the goal is attained, so that the patient achieves some measure of self care.

Resources

Resources available to handle problems of chronic disease vary considerably from community to community. Some areas have more long-term care facilities available than do others. Many areas of the country have no hospital beds specifically assigned to care for patients with chronic diseases, so that patients are maintained for weeks or months in a regular general hospital where few of the needed special services may be available.

One of the great problems existing throughout the country concerns the question of nursing homes. Not only is there a dearth of these facilities, but a substantial number fail to provide a reasonable level of care. Many nursing homes rely on nursing assistants to look after their patients, and far too few have engaged the services of other professional personnel, such as physical therapists. Often they are merely custodial institutions, providing little in the way of health care. Nevertheless, costs of care in nursing homes are rising rapidly. Some now charge as much as it used to cost for care in a general hospital, although it must be admitted that many of these homes now provide for a greater variety of health care services than was previously the case. However, more than half of all nursing-home patients today are supported by welfare payments, which are generally very low.

Considerable numbers of chronic disease patients remain in hospitals far beyond the time when they need such expensive services. Sometimes, of course, hospitalization is continued because there appears to be nowhere else for the patient to go. There may be no nursing-home bed available, or the patient may not have an adequate home. If the patient can be discharged to his home, he frequently needs home health services. While it is true that home care services have increased in recent years, in many communities these are still either nonexistent or the extent of services available is limited. A home care program needs to provide not only for medical and nursing services, but for physical, occupational and speech therapy, social and nutritional services and homemaker services.

Perhaps the greatest difficulty existing today in the provision of chronic disease services revolves around the availability of health manpower. This is in short supply in most sections of the country. Not only must we increase the supply of health manpower knowledgeable and interested in gerontology, but we must learn how to make better use of that which we now have. We must also learn how to utilize subprofessional personnel to assume some of the tasks which professional personnel are now performing.

Prevention and Control

Unlike many communicable diseases, the chronic diseases cannot, in general, be prevented by a simple immunization or by other prophylactic methods. Even here there are some exceptions, notably in the case of rheumatic fever, which may be prevented by early thorough treatment of streptococcal sore throat; but such examples, of course, are exceptions. Using our current state of knowledge, most chronic diseases cannot be prevented (primary prevention). On the other hand, with early detection and treatment, much can be done to prevent complications from occurring and leading to worsening of the patient's condition (secondary prevention). Certainly, a great deal can be done to limit the patient's disability and to provide him with rehabilitation measures which will enable him to carry on his everyday activities (tertiary prevention). In addition, as is true of many diseases, early detection may well play a key role in preventing disability from occurring at all, in retarding its development or in prolonging life.

On the other hand, many difficulties stand in the way of an effective program to control chronic diseases. One of these problems is the tremendous and continual rise in costs involved in diagnosis and treatment, added to which are the problems concerning inadequacy and inequitable distribution of health manpower and facilities to cope with the situation. These subjects are dealt with at more length in other chapters.

Another difficulty involves the gradual and often insidious onset of many chronic diseases, so that the patient is not motivated to seek medical advice until the disease is well advanced. Herein lies one of the advantages inherent in regular health examinations, particularly in persons 40 years of age and over.

Periodic Health Examinations

While there may be some disagreement among authorities as to the proper age at which regular examinations should be performed, there is little argument that, at least by age 40, an annual examination is desirable. This examination should include a medical history, a complete physical examination, the performance of certain laboratory tests and time set aside for interpretation of the results of the examination to the patient, followed by appropriate counselling and guidance. Among the important laboratory procedures which should be carried out are hemoglobin and blood sugar determinations, urinalysis, electrocardiogram, chest x-ray study and cervical cytologic examination. It can be anticipated that least one abnormality will be found in about 30% of persons examined. Among the commoner findings are obesity, hypertension, rectal polyps and anemia.

It should be stated that the value of periodic health examinations has been questioned by some authorities. In particular, doubts have been raised concerning the effective yield from such examinations. Furthermore, the desirability of using the limited health manpower currently available for the periodic examination rather than for the care of persons who exhibit obvious evidence of disease has been questioned. As time-savers in the periodic examination, the automated screening devices and self-administered history (Cornell Medical Index) may be of value.

Other Facets of Chronic Disease Control

Early Detection. The advantages of early case finding are obvious. Studies have revealed, for example, that of every 100 persons over the age of 40 tested for glaucoma, two will be found to have the disease, in whom it was previously unsuspected. Similarly, one person of every 100 over the age of 25 will be found to have previously unknown diabetes. The only possible danger is that if the patient is exposed to a battery of screening tests which reveal no abnormalities, he may feel that he is quite free of disease and, therefore, may not see the wisdom of a complete examination. Thus, screening tests require careful interpretation, so that the patient will understand that these tests are not a substitute for a complete examination.

Progressive Patient Care. A high percentage of patients with chronic disease will require periods of care in a general hospital, in a chronic disease hospital, or in a nursing home. On the other hand, many can be taken care of at home, if adequate health services can be made available at home to assist the patient, or someone on his behalf, to provide care. Such services may include nursing, physical therapy, homemaker service, and visits from a social worker.

Irrespective of what particular service is rendered the patient at any time, it is essential that the patient's physician insure that adequate continuity of care is preserved and that there is sufficient flexibility to permit the patient to be easily moved from one level of care to another as the occasion demands. This should apply to the medically indigent as well as the private patient.

Rehabilitation. Many patients, in fact the majority, with chronic diseases can be helped to become completely or partially self supporting, or at least to take care of their own personal needs rather than to be totally dependent upon relatives or friends. Aside from the obvious benefits of this rehabilitation process, the psychologic advantages to the patient, his relatives, and the community are great. Many patients can be returned to work, sometimes on a reduced schedule, or a less taxing job may be found suitable for both the patient and for management. The psychiatric aspects of rehabilitation are so important and obvious that perhaps it seems superfluous to mention them. Nevertheless, in practice they are often forgotten. Many a patient suffering from chronic disabling illness, not working, and dependent upon others for support, physically and financially, may feel that life is hardly worth living. Social service is essential under these conditions; the patient must have some meaningful activity, occupational, recreational, social or other, and will need a good deal of supportive therapy.

Cardiovascular Diseases

Diseases of the heart and blood vessels constitute the leading cause of death and disabling illness in the United States; they are responsible for approximately 50% of all deaths at the present time. In 1900, they accounted for only 20% of all deaths. This increase is primarily due to the increasing percentage of older persons in the population. At a matter of fact, if statistical allowance is made for this change in age distribution, it is found that the death rate from this group of causes has declined since 1930, particularly in persons under the age of 45 years. This, in turn, is due largely to the decreasing mortality from rheumatic heart disease. Similar progress has not been made in connection with arteriosclerosis and hypertension, which are particularly common as age advances. The mortality rates of coronary artery disease have, in fact, slightly increased.

Congenital Heart Disease. The incidence of congenital heart disease in newborn babies is approximately three per thousand live births. More than half die in the first year of life, the majority succumbing within a few days following birth.

A preventive measure that can be taken against one type involves the avoidance of rubella infection by pregnant women during the first trimester of pregnancy. For this reason, purposeful exposure of little girls to rubella is an important preventive technique. Should a pregnant woman become exposed, gamma globulin can be given.

In addition to primary prevention, modern surgical techniques have greatly improved the prognosis for persons with congenital heart disease. However, early case finding is essential, and children who exhibit symptoms such as cyanosis or breathlessness should be referred for an expert evaluation.

Infectious Heart Disease. Heart disease as a complication of diphtheria, once not uncommon, is now a rarity, and syphilitic heart disease has become much less frequent as a result of measures taken to control syphilis.

Rheumatic heart disease is the most common type of infectious heart disease; however, it, too, may be prevented by prompt and thorough antibiotic treatment of streptococcal infections. Furthermore, prophylactic penicillin is also effective in preventing recurrent episodes in persons already afflicted with rheumatic fever. Similarly, bacterial endocarditis may be prevented by judicious use of antibiotics in patients with rheumatic fever or congenital heart disease. This is particularly important if dental surgery or nose and throat operations are to be performed on such a patient.

Rheumatic fever has been clearly shown to occur most commonly among families of the low-income group living in overcrowded homes, especially in the families having a previously affected child. Careful surveillance of these families is therefore desirable. This is particularly important in light of the fact that rheumatic fever often produces vague symptoms which are frequently overlooked; damage to the heart, nevertheless, may occur.

Arteriosclerosis and Hypertension. While our knowledge concerning the exact etiologic factors involved in the development of arteriosclerosis and coronary artery disease leaves much to be desired, it has long been known that, in arteriosclerosis, deposits of fat, including cholesterol, are found in the affected blood vessels. Furthermore, it has been demonstrated that patients with coronary artery disease, in general, have elevated blood cholesterol levels. It is as a result of these facts that hope of affecting the disease, at least to some extent, through control of fat metabolism has developed. However, it is by no means certain that reduction of cholesterol intake will prevent high cholesterol blood levels since the body synthesizes cholesterol through ordinary metabolic processes. Moreover, hypertension and cigarette smoking both appear to predispose patients to the development of coronary artery disease.

Three factors appear to be most important in the production of hypertension; these are:

1. A strong familial tendency
2. Obesity
3. Personality

When hypertension occurs in an adult, it may almost be taken for granted that the children will be similarly affected. In instances of obesity, weight reduction alone may effect a lowering of the blood pressure, while the sharp, albeit temporary, increases in blood pressure that occur as a result of psychic stresses, such as anxiety or fear, are well recognized. From this well-known fact,

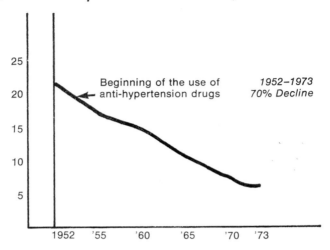

Source: The Killers and Cripplers. National Health Education Committee, 1976.

Fig. 12.   Decline in the Death Rate From Hypertensive Heart Disease.

it has been postulated that hypertension may be due, in part, to repeated psychic traumata occurring over long periods. However, much more research is necessary before this hypothesis can be accepted.

Prevention. Obviously, in the light of our present lack of knowledge, primary prevention of arteriosclerosis and hypertension does not seem practicable. However, measures can be taken to prevent disability and premature death. For this purpose, early diagnosis is essential. Proper management of patients with hypertension or arteriosclerotic heart disease includes dietary and occupational adjustment, together with emotional support, as well as consideration of the use of drugs and salt restriction. Such steps may not only prolong the patient's life but may also make him much happier.

Cancer

While cancer occurs most commonly among those in middle and old age, it must nevertheless be recognized that mortality from cancer is second only to accidents as a cause of death in children between the ages of 1 and 15 years. Cancer is now the second leading cause of death in the United States, being responsible for more than 15% of all deaths. While much of the increased incidence appears to be the result of changes in age distribution, some cancers appear to have actu-

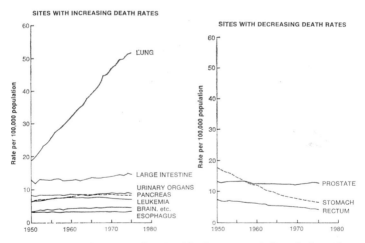

Source: National Center for Health Statistics: Selected data from Division of Vital Statistics

Fig. 13. Age-adjusted death rates for white males for leading sites of malignant neoplasms: United States, 1950–75.

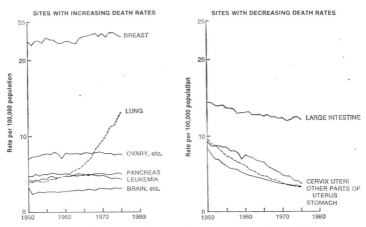

Source: National Center for Health Statistics: Selected data from Division of Vital Statistics

Fig. 14. Age-adjusted death rates for white females for leading sites of malignant neoplasms: United States, 1950–75.

ally become more common, for example, lung cancer. There is no question that even in these cases at least part of the increase is due to improvements in diagnosis and reporting.

The total incidence of cancer is similar in the two sexes, but half of all female cancer occurs in the breast and genitals, while half of all cancer in males originates in the digestive system. Cancers of the lung and larynx are much more common in the male than in the female. Furthermore, as one descends the socioeconomic ladder, cancer incidence generally appears to rise. Mortality is lower in women, probably because the most common female cancers are more accessible than are those in the male, more likely to be noticed and more likely, therefore, to be detected and treated at an early date.

Etiologic Factors. While the exact cause of cancer is not known, some light has been shed on factors involved in the development of at least a number of cancers.

1. *Genetic factors.* There is strong evidence of a familial tendency to a number of cancers, including carcinoma of the breast. Breast cancer is found more commonly in daughters of women who have had a similar cancer.

2. *Carcinogens.* A number of chemicals used in industrial processes appear to lead to cancer when exposure occurs over prolonged periods. Radioactive emanations are also capable of causing cancer; leukemia is considerably more prevalent among radiologists than in the general population.

3. *Pre-cancerous lesions.* A number of apparently benign lesions may become the site of cancer; examples include intestinal polyposis and adenoma of the thyroid.

4. *Chronic irritation.* Cancer of the tongue is often associated with the presence of jagged teeth; pipe smokers may develop cancer of the lip; cancer of the skin may occur in farmers exposed continually to ultraviolet rays of the sun.

5. *Cigarette smoking.* Clear evidence of the association between lung cancer and cigarette smoking has accumulated.

Prevention. Obviously, opportunities for primary prevention of cancer are presently limited. However, reduction or elimination of exposure to industrial carcinogens provides a real opportunity to reduce some cancer. Reduction or elimination of smoking, albeit difficult of achievement, would contribute materially to a decrease in lung cancer. Similarly, consideration must be given to the removal of pre-cancerous lesions.

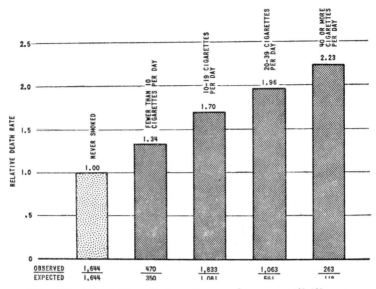

Fig. 15. Mortality of cigarette smokers, age 50-59 years: ratios of observed to expected numbers of deaths by daily cigarette consumption. (Hammond: The effects of smoking. *Scientific American*, Vol. 207.)

Many more possibilities for control exist under the heading of secondary prevention. For successful prevention of further progression of the disease, however, early detection is absolutely essential. In fact, in some types of cancer such as skin cancer, early detection, followed by appropriate treatment, will often result in a complete cure. Nowhere are early diagnosis and treatment more important than in cancer, where any delay may lead to premature death of the patient as a result of spread to the lymph nodes, blood vessels and other organs.

Cancer Detection. Among the important steps that should be taken to provide for early case finding is patient education concerning some of the early signs of cancer which should lead the patient to see his physician. Female patients may be taught self-examination of the breasts. Routine cervical smears from women age 40 and over are very important; in fact, some authorities recommend that this be performed annually from age 30. Routine chest x-ray films may reveal evidence of lung cancer, while occult blood in the stools may lead the physician to suspect cancer of the digestive tract.

Once cancer has been detected, immediate thorough treatment is indicated. Rehabilitation services for cancer patients should include emotional rehabilitation. Indeed, this may be the most important part of the therapy.

Chronic Respiratory Disease

Included under this heading are such conditions as bronchitis and emphysema, asthma and bronchiectasis. These diseases are responsible for substantial disability due to impairment of respiratory function. While deaths from pneumonia and tuberculosis have declined in the past half-century, mortality from bronchitis and emphysema has risen because, at least partially, those persons who used to succumb to diseases such as tuberculosis now survive, still retaining respiratory impairment, only to die eventually of emphysema.

Interest in these chronic respiratory diseases has heightened in recent years, again due, in some measure, to the decline in tuberculosis mortality. For example, the National Tuberculosis Association has, in recent years, embarked on a campaign against the chronic respiratory diseases in addition to its more traditional role of fighting tuberculosis.

The chronic respiratory diseases produce an impairment of respiratory function which increases with advancing age, and mortality rates are much higher in older age groups. Furthermore, there is both a seasonal fluctuation (mortality generally being higher in the winter months) and an urban-rural variation (mortality tending to be higher in cities). It also appears that the incidence increases with the degree of poverty. Air pollution and cigarette smoking have both been incriminated as important factors in the production of these diseases and in their aggravation. Genetic and allergic factors may also be important as in asthma.

Primary prevention will be dependent upon more information being obtained as to the relative importance of these various factors; however, air pollution, cigarette smoking, and occupational exposure can be attacked now. Early diagnosis, followed by thorough treatment and rehabilitation, may do much to reduce death and disability from these diseases.

Arthritis

The various forms of arthritis (infections, rheumatoid, osteoarthritis and gout) may be characterized as producing prolonged disability, but seldom death. It has been estimated that there are more than 24 million persons in the United States with arthritis and that some 25% have disability of sufficient degree to limit their activities considerably. The prevalence of arthritis and the extent of disability, in general, increase with age. From the point of view of the patients, these diseases cause pain, limitation of mobility, disability and loss of time from work.

1. *Infectious arthritis* usually involves a single joint and may be caused by many different organisms, including the gonococcus. Control of gonorrhea would

therefore essentially eliminate gonococcal arthritis. Tuberculous arthritis has been almost eliminated in the United States as a result of the pasteurization of milk.

2. *Rheumatoid arthritis* most commonly affects young adults, usually in their 30's, and is much more frequent in women than in men; however, once it becomes established it continues, as a rule, throughout life, often leading to deformity and profound disability. It is most prevalent among poorer families and appears to have a familial tendency in some cases. The most important tools used in limiting serious disability are physical therapy and the use of orthopedic devices.

3. *Osteoarthritis* is a degenerative disease of the joints occurring with increasing frequency as age advances. It occurs particularly in weight-bearing joints such as the knees. Obesity may be a factor, probably by producing faulty posture. As in rheumatoid arthritis, physical therapy offers the greatest hope for limitation of disability.

4. *Gout*, a painful, inflammatory disease, occurs most commonly in men. It has a strong hereditary tendency and also appears to be related to alcoholic and dietary excesses. Besides treatment with colchicine, meat and alcohol intake should be limited.

Patients with arthritis benefit greatly from progressive rehabilitation provided, when needed, in the rehabilitation unit of a community general hospital.

Diabetes

Diabetes affects approximately 5% of the population and currently ranks as the sixth leading cause of death in the United States. Women are 50% more likely than men to have diabetes, and it is more common among black people and the poor. It is also more frequent in obese individuals, and the incidence of dia-

Characteristic	All ages	Under 17 years	17–44 years	45–64 years	65 years and over	All ages	Under 17 years	17–44 years	45–64 years	65 years and over
	Prevalence of conditions in thousands					Number per 1,000 persons				
Total[1]	24,573	137	3,855	11,065	9,517	116.7	2.2	45.5	255.8	436.6
Sex										
Male	8,475	47	1,332	4,067	3,028	83.4	1.5	32.5	197.1	337.9
Female	16,098	89	2,523	6,997	6,489	147.7	3.0	57.7	309.3	505.5
Color										
White	21,794	116	3,388	9,753	8,538	119.2	2.3	46.1	251.6	431.9
All other	2,779	*21	466	1,312	980	100.0	*2.1	41.7	291.8	482.8
Family income										
Under $5,000	6,336	*18	548	1,901	3,868	218.6	*2.7	56.0	389.9	497.5
$5,000–$9,999	5,747	*24	778	2,414	2,531	135.1	*2.0	47.5	307.8	412.5
$10,000–$14,999	4,046	*30	926	2,155	936	91.0	*2.1	47.4	253.4	405.5
$15,000 or more	6,012	49	1,393	3,554	1,017	79.3	2.2	42.0	203.7	385.1
Education of head of family										
Less than 9 years	8,761	*19	598	3,464	4,680	211.4	*1.9	56.0	321.9	468.2
9–11 years	4,055	*32	609	1,988	1,426	123.5	*3.1	50.9	267.5	442.6
12 years	6,201	50	1,380	3,060	1,711	90.5	2.3	46.2	234.8	403.8
13–15 years	2,507	*15	623	1,137	732	82.0	*1.7	41.2	226.7	420.4
16 years or more	2,599	*21	601	1,224	754	75.6	*2.1	37.1	197.0	376.6

Place of residence										
SMSA	15,752	89	2,586	7,185	5,892	109.2	2.2	43.6	240.0	424.9
Central city	7,182	35	1,037	3,146	2,964	116.9	2.1	41.5	248.6	425.9
Not central city	8,570	55	1,549	4,039	2,927	103.5	2.3	45.2	233.7	423.8
Outside SMSA	8,821	47	1,268	3,880	3,626	132.8	2.4	49.9	291.4	457.1
Nonfarm	7,829	38	1,156	3,373	3,261	130.7	2.1	49.7	288.7	459.9
Farm	992	*9	112	506	365	151.7	*4.7	52.0	310.4	433.5
Geographic region										
Northeast	5,254	*32	743	2,405	2,074	108.1	*2.4	39.0	219.2	405.3
North Central	6,782	42	1,165	2,974	2,601	120.6	2.6	51.2	261.8	439.1
South	8,276	39	1,202	3,782	3,252	122.5	1.9	44.8	278.7	459.6
West	4,260	*23	744	1,903	1,591	111.4	*2.1	46.2	258.9	432.1

[1] Includes unknown income and education.

[Data are based on household interviews of the civilian noninstitutionalized population.]

NOTE: When a figure is shown with an asterisk, it is presented only for the purpose of combining with other cells. An estimate will have a relative standard error less than 30 percent when the aggregate is at least 35,000.

Source: From the Health Interview Survey, United States, 1976.

Fig. 16. Prevalence of arthritis, not elsewhere classifiable, and number per 1,000 persons, by age and selected characteristics: United States, 1976.

betes rises rapidly with advancing age. The prolonged life expectancy made possible by insulin has revealed many previously unrecognized complications of the disease, such as, blindness, kidney, and cardiovascular diseases. In the United States there are some 4,500,000 known diabetics with perhaps an equal number of individuals who have the disease but are unaware of it.

Prevention. Consideration should be given to avoidance of marriage between diabetics, because of the strong probability that diabetes will appear in their offspring. If the marriage does occur, consideration should be given to the use of birth control measures. At least the marital partners need to be aware of the strong possibility that their offspring will have diabetes, and be prepared for this eventuality.

Dietary control is also important among families with a diabetic history. In fact, blood sugar may well be reduced when weight reduction is brought about.

Detection of diabetes should be carried out as early as possible. Blood-testing in 100 persons over the age of 25 years will usually uncover one previously unknown diabetic. Emphasis in case finding should be placed on detecting the disease in families of known diabetics. Therefore, family members should have regular routine urinalysis and blood sugar determination.

Early discovery of diabetes followed by proper management of the patient, using dietary control supplemented as necessary by insulin, with emphasis upon the avoidance of infections and the practice of good foot hygiene, will play an important part in minimizing the danger of complications and ensuring maximum life expectancy.

Loss of Vision

Persons having a visual acuity of 20/200 or less (with corrective glasses) are usually classified as blind.

It has been estimated that using this definition of blindness there are approximately two blind persons per 1,000 population in the United States. The total number of blind persons in this country numbers about 400,000. Among the commonest causes of blindness and less severe loss of vision are senile cataract, glaucoma, infectious diseases and diabetes.

Prevention. Some of the once-common causes of blindness have almost disappeared as a result of preventive measures. For example, prophylactic silver nitrate in the eyes of newborn infants has almost eliminated ophthalmia neonatorum due to gonorrhea. Similarly, blindness resulting from congenital syphilis has been prevented by thorough treatment of pregnant women found to be infected. Retrolental fibroplasia, which occurred particularly in premature babies given high concentrations of oxyegn, now rarely occurs since its cause has been discovered.

While primary prevention of loss of vision due to most of the remaining causes of visual defects is often not possible, secondary and tertiary prevention is feasible in many cases. However, early case detection is essential. This often requires vision screening in children, often in preschool children but certainly in children of elementary school age. Strabismus found early may be relatively easy to correct if detected and treated before the child is 6 years old. Finding of visual defects among children, followed by corrective steps, including the provision of glasses where required, is an important secondary preventive measure as well as contributing materially to the child's progress at school.

Glaucoma is a condition which most commonly begins at or over age 40, often coming on insidiously and producing considerable loss of vision before the patient is aware of the change. This fact is of great importance when it is realized that approximately 2% of persons over the age of 40 are found to have glaucoma; if the patient is treated early by medical or surgical means, much blindness may be prevented. Routine tonometry in persons over 40 years is therefore an important preventive measure.

Cataracts also occur most commonly in middle or old age and are the most common cause of blindness in the United States. Early case finding, followed by surgical removal of the lens, accompanied by the use of appropriate glasses can help restore useful vision in most cases.

Special classes for blind children and vocational rehabilitation for blind adolescents and adults together with necessary counselling services are important and desirable community programs.

Loss of Hearing

There are two types of deafness: conductive and perceptive. Conductive deafness is due to faulty transmission of sound to the cochlear nerve endings; perceptive deafness results from abnormalities beginning with the cochlear nerve endings and ending in the hearing center in the brain.

Deafness may be congenital or acquired and may be caused by infections, or physical or chemical agents. Some of the causes are syphilis, German measles (occurring in pregnant women and producing deafness in the child), wax, foreign bodies, streptomycin and quinine. Deafness may also result from brain or vascular disorders and from environmental factors, related particularly to the intensity of sounds. Prolonged exposure to high intensity levels will produce cochlear damage.

Prevention. If two otosclerotic persons marry, a high proportion of their offspring will have otosclerosis; genetic counselling is therefore important under these circumstances. Prevention of German measles in pregnant women and thorough treatment of syphilis will prevent deafness from these causes. Infections of the ear should be thoroughly treated as soon as detected, and care should be exercised in the use of drugs such as streptomycin and quinine. The patient should be maintained under constant surveillance. In the working environment, muffling devices and improved engineering can do much to cut down decibel levels.

Other than the use of antibiotics in the treatment of otitis media, opportunities for primary prevention are very limited and are related to the etiologic factors outlined above. However, early case finding followed by appropriate corrective measures may do much to reduce hearing loss and to otherwise assist patients in minimizing disability. Screening programs, e.g., use of the audiometer among school children, will uncover many cases of hearing loss. The provision of hearing aids must always be accompanied by training in their use. Special classes for deaf children and vocational rehabilitation for adolescents and adults are important community services.

REFERENCES

Breslow, L.: Chronic Disease and Disability in Adults, in *Preventive Medicine and Public Health,* Sartwell, Maxcy, and Rosenau, 10th Ed., New York, Appleton-Century-Crofts, Inc., 1973.

————— : Prevention and control of chronic disease. Periodic health examinations and multiple screening. Amer. J. Publ. Health 49:1149, 1959.

Commission on Chronic Illness: *Chronic Illness in the United States,* Vol. 4, Chronic Illness in a Large City, Cambridge, Mass., Harvard University Press for the Commonwealth Fund, 1957.

Comprehensive Care Services in Your Community, U.S. Department of HEW, 1967.

Dorn, H. F., and Cutler, S. J.: *Morbidity from Cancer in the United States*, Public Health Monograph 56, Washington D.C., U.S. Dept. of Health, Education and Welfare, 1959.

Kilbourne, E. D., and Smillie, W. G.: *Human Ecology and Public Health*, 4th Ed., New York, The Macmillan Co., 1969.

National Conference on Chronic Disease, Preventive Aspects, Chicago, 1951, Report of the Commission on Chronic Illness, Raleigh, N.C., Health Publications Institute, 1952.

Report of the National Commission on Diabetes to the Congress of the United States, Washington, D. C., Vol. 1, December 1975.

Royal College of Physicians:*Smoking and Health*, London, Pitman Pub. Corp., 1962.

Smoking and Health, Report of the Advisory Committee to the Surgeon General of the Public Health Service, PHS Publication No. 1103, Washington, D.C., Government Printing Office, 1964.

The Present Health System Defined, by Anne R. Somers. Presented at National Health Forum, 1967.

Wilner, D. M., Walkley, R. P., and O'Neill, E. J.: *Introduction to Public Health*, New York, The Macmillan Co., 1978.

Chapter **5**

Geriatrics

In 1900 only 4% of the population of the United States was 65 years of age or older. Today 11% of the population, or more than 20 million people are over 65 years of age. By the year 2020 this could increase to 25%. Average life expectancy increased from 47 years in 1900 to 73 years in 1977. It should be noted that while the expectation of life at birth has increased steadily, the expectation at 65 years has changed little having risen by only 4 years since the turn of the century.

In January 1971, one-half of the elderly or over 10 million people, lived on less than $10 a day. At least 30% of the elderly live in substandard housing. Eighty-six per cent have chronic health problems of varying degrees. A serious illness may mean instant poverty. While a large number of older people in America are poor by Government definition, many more barely manage to survive. Over one-half lack food and essential drugs.

Old women tend to fare worse than old men. Their average life expectancy is 7 years longer than men and two-thirds of all older women are widows and are likely to end up alone.

At any one time, some 95% of the elderly live in the community and only some 5% are in nursing homes, chronic disease hospitals and other institutions. More than 90% are fully ambulatory and move about freely on their own.

The elderly account for approximately one-fourth of the Nation's health expenditures because of their greater need for medical services and their costlier illnesses. Older patients require more of the physician's time, more frequent hospital admissions and longer hospital stays. They are the main users of long-term care facilities and home health agencies; they consume 25% of all drugs consumed in the United States. Their leading causes of death are heart disease, cancer, stroke and accidents, but the care of chronic conditions constitutes the bulk of their physical health problems.

Caring for the medical needs of older people requires knowledge of the special ways by which illness manifests itself in this age group. For example, acute illness may not present the classic signs of fever and elevated blood count found in younger people. Many physicians are not keen on working with old people, particularly those who are senile. Medical schools find them "uninteresting." Hospitals funnel them into nursing homes, mental hospitals, and chronic disease institutions. Those who remain at home have serious difficulties in securing medical, social, and psychiatric services.

Older patients often have difficulties when they need hospitalization unless they have a regular doctor or a sizeable income. A significant number appear at the hospital emergency room and frequently have a long wait before securing examination, treatment, or admission. Tranquilizers and antidepressant drugs are extensively used by old people, particularly those suffering agitation, anxiety and depression. These drugs are often given as much for the tranquility of the institution as for the comfort of the patient.

Old age has the potential for being an interesting and emotionally satisfying period of life, but this potential is endangered by many forces, such as loss of physical health or the death of relatives or friends. Crises of all kinds must be met, sometimes simultaneously—retirement, widowhood, illness, changes in bodily appearance, and a lowered standard of living. Well over 50% of nursing home patients have evidence of mental impairment.

Prejudices and misconceptions concerning age has caused society to treat old people in ways which are totally unjustified. If we insist that there is a group of people who, on a fixed calendar basis cease to be people and become unintelligent, asexual, unemployable, and psychotic, then persons who are so designated will be under pressure to act and to be treated accordingly. Generalizing from a person's chronologic age to his or her ability to perform certain types of activities is likely to prove dangerous. Furthermore, there is a greater degree of homogeneity of physical and mental abilities in a group of 12 year olds than there is in a group of 70 year olds.

Psychological and Biological Changes

Each human being ages at his own rate and in his own way. The nursing home patient—bedridden with a stroke, paralysis, and senility—may be aged 60, 70, 85 or 95. Many older people seem quite undiminished in their physical powers. The rate and pace of individual aging largely depends on genetic inheritance, nutrition and diet, physical activity, and psychosocial factors.

Actually, decline generally begins at age 30 and continues for the rest of the individual's life. Metabolic rate, cardiac output, kidney function, and breathing capacity usually reach their peak at age 30 and decline steadily thereafter, although not at the same rate. The body subtly and inconspicuously loses its resilience; muscles lose their tone; tissues and organs become rigid, less elastic and less adaptable to stress. Thus, blows, jerks, and falls which younger persons brush aside often cause serious injury in older persons.

The various parts of the body contain less fluid as they age; joints stiffen; chest tissues tighten making breathing more difficult. The skin dries and impairs the ability of the body to control surface temperature through perspiration.

The older person who survives a medical crisis will recover from it more slowly. On the average, a wound which heals in 31 days in a youth of 20 takes 100 days to heal in a man of 60.

Physical activity and fitness is perhaps the best documented of all factors that appear to produce long life. A study of the effects of a program of graduated but heavy exercise on a group of sedentary middle-aged men found substantial improvements in the efficiency of a number of physiological functions that ordinarily decline with age. It was found that exercise brought a lower heart rate, greater pumping capacity of the heart, lower blood pressure, greater lung capacity and more efficient fat metabolism. Numerous studies have documented the positive benefits of regular exercise on the heart and lungs.

Socioeconomic Changes

By the age of 65, most workers are retired and endeavoring to adjust to a new life style centered around rest and leisure. At that same time, there is usually entitlement to some new rights such as social security benefits, Medicare, and perhaps some reduced costs for public transportation and amusements.

At the same time, however, the user's income is severely cut and further depleted by inflation. He gives up productive work and his word carries less weight with grown children; in fact, he must often accept a position of dependence on them. Older persons face a curious dilemma. Medical science and high living standards give millions of people a healthy old age. Yet, our society's posture toward these people is appropriate only for those who are about to die.

Demographic and Cultural Changes

Both the numbers and proportion of older people in the American population have been on the increase. In 1900 some 3 million Americans were aged 65 and over; today, the figure exceeds 20 million. Within the next 50 years, the number will double to more than 40 million. The 1970 Census found that about 1/3 of the 21 million older persons were aged 75 or older. Women live substantially longer than men. The male life expectancy at birth is currently 69 years, the female 77 years.

In 1900, some 40% of American people lived in urban areas. Today this figure exceeds 70%. Older people are over-represented in the central sections of our larger cities and less so in the booming suburban areas.

American society has tended to deprive the older person of the one role he has had in most traditional cultures, namely the role of the elder statesman who epitomizes social stability and continuity with the past. A society which cherishes the present and future has little need for someone to embody the past.

Adjustment to Aging

The old person must first admit that age brings limitations to his physical and mental abilities. Unfortunately, many deny that age has brought about any changes; they often work harder, hurl themselves into new activities, and try to look younger. Others attribute changes to sickness rather than age.

Once he has accepted the limitations brought about by old age, the elderly person must trim down his world to match the facts. He must learn to delegate some responsibilities to others and perhaps move to a smaller dwelling.

The older person needs to find new ways to fulfill his physical, emotional, and economical needs. The man who is retiring must endeavor to find an adequate income; he may have to seek new friends to replace those at work and new activities should be explored.

Maladjustment

Anxiety often becomes chronic in old age. The old person may experience anxiety as a vague but persistent dread, which may be accompanied by muscular tension, restlessness, and rapid heart rate. This anxiety is often rooted in a fear of growing old.

Sleep disturbances of all kinds are common. It has been estimated that approximately one-third of all old people habitually use sleeping pills.

Recurrent periods of depression are perhaps the most common neuroses of old age. The elderly often feel discouraged, worried, useless, and bored.

Hypochondriasis is common in old people, particularly in women. Cataloguing pains and symptoms is a frequent preoccupation of old persons and is often designed to elicit sympathy and attention.

Health Needs

Health care needs of older people are substantially different from those of other segments of the population. The major challenge for older persons is to learn to live with debilitating chronic illness. Older people also constitute approximately one-third of all patients in public mental hospitals. The elderly are, furthermore, more likely to be malnourished and face a problem almost unique to them—a lack of high quality nursing homes and other long-term care facilities.

Worries about health care and the cost of health rank at the top of most surveys of older people's opinions about their needs and problems. Some 80% of older persons are afflicted so some degree by one or more chronic conditions such as arthritis, rheumatism, heart disease, high blood pressure, diabetes, chronic bronchitis, or ulcers. This chronic illness severely limits the activities of about one-half of all Americans aged 65 and over. Managing these chronic diseases consumes much time and often requires strenuous effort. For example, heart patients may move to a one story house; arthritics may rearrange furniture for maximum convenience. Many older people, however, succumb to the limitations of chronic illness because they lack the judgment or the assistance to make the necessary adjustments.

Medicare can work reasonably well for an older person stricken with an illness which requires a fairly short stay in a hospital. However, it works less well when the person is afflicted with a long-term chronic illness. On the average, Medicare pays less than half each older person's medical care bill. Most of this is due to the fact that many expenditures are excluded from the Medicare program. Examples are, prescription drugs, dental care, eye glasses, hearing aids, foot and eye care, long-term care in nursing homes without prior hospitalization, and most psychiatric care as well as transportation required to secure health care services. In addition, the fees and deductibles older people are required to pay under Medicare have doubled since the program was initiated in 1965. Finally, inflation has driven up the cost of medical care services. In general, these costs have been increasing twice as fast as the cost of living.

Clearly, some of these costs have been absorbed by the Medicaid program, but since this is a state operated activity (with Federal financial support), the degree to which these costs are absorbed varies from State to State.

It is also pertinent to point out that, as a general rule, physicians do not usually show the same degree of interest in providing medical care services to older persons with chronic diseases as they do to a younger person suffering from an acute illness. There is, in fact, a tendency for many nursing home patients to be essentially left to their own devices with such care as is provided being supplied by a nursing assistant supported by occasional visits from a registered nurse and by far less frequent visits by the doctor.

Prevention

An effective preventive program for older people must obviously begin before age 65. Such a program should include effective health education, a life-long practice of regular medical check-ups, and measures to facilitate early detection of disease with appropriate follow-up. These preventive needs are largely unmet, at least in most segments of society. Common screening tests to determine symptoms of some diseases are coming into wider use. Multiphasic screening in which several conditions may be detected at "one sitting" has been instituted in recent years but follow-up and referral leave much to be desired.

Mental health services for older people are generally meager. The elderly either receive no psychiatric attenten or they are committed for long periods of time, often for life, to institutions which offer little more than custodial care. While older persons account for almost one-third of public mental hospital patients, they account for only 2% of the patients in psychiatric outpatient clinics.

Some 5% of the elderly live in institutions. Some of these institutions provide excellent care; others are grossly deficient. They frequently do not provide the level of care they say they provide. The staff may be poorly trained and the facilities and services offered may be quite inadequate. Mentally ill people languish in nursing homes; physically ill older people live in mental hospitals. The average age of nursing home residents is 78 and two-thirds are women. Almost 90% of those persons entering nursing homes die in them. Good care in nursing homes is expensive and is available in only a limited number of homes. If the individual in need of nursing home care has moderate resources, he must first exhaust them and then apply for Medicaid after he has become poor.

REFERENCES

Manney, James D., Jr.: *Aging in American Society*, Ann Arbor, Michigan, Institute of Gerontology (Sponsored jointly by University of Michigan and Wayne State University), 1975.

Reissman, F.: *Older Persons—Unused Resources for Unmet Needs*, Beverly Hills, California, Sage, 1977.

Butler, R.: *Why Survive—Being Old in America*, New York, Harper & Row, 1975.

4

Chapter 6

Medical Sociology

Sociologists have long been interested in the distribution of illness and the factors which lead to its selective occurrence. Increasingly, sociologic literature on disease distribution has dealt with such variables as age, sex, occupation, and income. However, increasing attention is now given to attitudes and behavior; sociologists are currently concerned with people's conception of their own health, their response to illness, and the many social and cultural differences which may impact on health and illness.

Sociologists are interested in determining the effect of social change and cultural patterns on the relationship between the patient and the health care provider and on the organization of health care systems. They are also concerned with patient responsibility and in the development of self-help groups, such as Alcoholics Anonymous. They study the consequences of using nurse practitioners as an alternative to physicians in some areas, and the influence of different financing mechanisms or organization frameworks on variations in hospital utilization, or on the extent of surgical treatment. They explore the manner by which physicians influence each other or affect the work of other health personnel.

Medical sociologists examine the effect of bureaucracy, professional rivalry, the division of labor, and decision making in hospital organization and operations. They study the relationships of community health agencies and the influence of those relationships on the development of health services. They examine into the use of health manpower and resources and the extent to which inappropriate utilization may occur.

Medical sociologists are interested in the effect of social stress and its relationship to diseases such as heart disease. They examine into methods for assessing behavior and assisting people to overcome problems. There is considerable interest in political influences in the health field; these include the extent to which special interests attempt to define medical priorities, obtain preferential legislation, or distort the delivery of health services.

The importance of medical sociology to the field of community health may be viewed from the vantage point of automobile accidents. These are the fourth leading cause of death in the United States and the most important cause of death between 15 and 35 years of age.

The causative agent is, of course, the automobile itself. Consequently, its structure and safety features have an important bearing on the occupant's susceptibility to an accident and the extent of injury when an accident occurs.

The environment includes the highway with its traffic control patterns, signs, lighting, and weather conditions. A sharp drop in highway mortality followed rapidly on the heels of the establishment of a 55-mile-per-hour speed limit.

Clearly, the characteristics of the host are important in the development of automobile accidents. The use of alcohol obviously looms large as a causative factor. A significant proportion of drivers killed in accidents have high blood alcohol levels. There is also substantial evidence that stress and anger may contribute to taking risks in driving which contribute to the possibility of injury or death.

Behavioral Science, Health and Disease

The concept of disease is applied in different ways. Narrowly speaking, it applies to a pathologic process which produces specific symptoms and signs. More generally, it refers to physical or behavioral deviations that produce problems either for the individual or for the community. Implicit in these broad definitions is a concept of normal health; however, the definition of health may differ in varying environments and cultures. Thus, in some cultures, an obese woman is an object of envy and desire. Epileptics may be regarded as having supernatural powers.

From the earliest times, man has sought relief from pain and discomfort. At first he looked to God and only later to man. The modern physician assesses the patient's condition compared to a norm, although it must be recognized that many of the standards he uses, even today, are quite tentative. Physicians may also have opposing views on the management of disease.

Such variability is inevitable in the presence of uncertain standards by which to measure the patient. What the physician does also depends upon his patient's and his community's expectations. Thus, a prescription may not be necessary for the patient's physical illness, but only for his emotional satisfaction. Much of medical practice involves helping people to conform more adequately to social rather than to physical standards.

Similarly, patients visit doctors for many reasons. Whether the patient even recognizes a problem depends on whether he has experienced a change which he views as troublesome. In other words, he has his own ideas as to what is "normal". These ideas are based on personal experience, cultural conditioning, and knowledge acquired during life.

Once he has recognized a problem, he may attribute it to being tired and overworked or having committed some wrong, or being possessed by evil spirits, or having been infected by a particular germ.

The doctor's views are molded by his professional training and experience; the patient's views are influenced by his need to cope with a particular problem and his social and cultural understanding of that problem.

It must be recognized that in the long run our wellbeing is less dependent on the sophistication of medical practice than on how we choose to live and what is done to our environment. Man has a remarkable biologic ability to adapt to his environment. Anthropologists have described a number of primitive groups that can sleep in the open in cold weather without clothes or blankets.

On the other hand, cultural patterns and ways of life give substance to the manner in which illness is perceived, expressed, and reacted to. The chronic alcoholic believes that only another alcoholic can understand his problems. Behaviors regarding smoking, the use of alcohol and other drugs, diet, exercise, and driving constitute major risk factors in heart disease, cancer, accidents, and liver cirrhosis. Group norms concerning smoking, drinking, standards of living, and sexual prac-

tices either predispose or protect adherents from risk
of disease. Indians may starve but they are reluctant to
kill their cattle. For those people considering the family
as of central importance, the hospital or nursing home
are threatening. People in some cultures may be unwilling to undergo pain and discomfort to achieve some
further protection from disease because they are
oriented to the present rather than the future. Public
health workers have often encountered difficulty in
changing people's diets because of social or religious
customs.

A person's lifestyle clearly has important implications
for his health. What we eat and drink, and how much,
the cigarette smoke we do or do not inhale, how fast
we drive, how much alcohol we consume, whether or
not we exercise regularly and whether or not we fasten
our seat belt all impact on our chances of increasing
our longevity.

Reaction to Health and Illness

Symptoms are differently perceived, evaluated, and
acted upon by different kinds of people and in different
social situations. Whether because of their earlier experiences, different training, different biologic sensitiv-
ity, or fear of the diagnosis, some persons make light of
symptoms and avoid seeking medical care. Others respond to a little pain and discomfort by readily seeking
care, securing release from work or other obligations,
and easily becoming dependent upon others.

The most frequent reason given for seeking a doctor
is the common cold. However, many people with colds
do not consult doctors and people who consult doctors
because of colds on one occasion may not do so on
another. It may well be that, in some instances, the
common cold is merely an excuse for visiting the physi-

cian in the desire to relieve the stress of a job which is disliked or an unhappy family situation. On the other hand, it is important to note that if the common cold as a justification became less viable, people would find other excuses to seek relief from their obligations.

Many studies have indicated that women report symptoms more frequently than men and use medical and psychiatric facilities more commonly. Reasons cited by investigators include—real differences in the prevalence of psychological disorders, women's lower threshold, differences between men and women in willingness to acknowledge the presence of symptoms, and psychobiologic differences between male and female.

Whether or not an individual seeks medical care may also depend on the accessibility of that care. Barriers may result from the location, economic impairments, bureaucratic harassment, social distance between patient and provider, or stigma associated with the ailment. It is clear, however, that persons are more likely to endeavor to take action for symptoms that in some way disrupt their usual functioning.

Variations in illness behavior in different societies are often quite obvious. For example, Koos observed that upper-class persons were more likely than lower-class persons to view themselves as ill when they had certain symptoms; they also more frequently would seek the doctor's advice. Saunders described the differences between English and Spanish-speaking people in the American Southwest in their attitudes and responses toward illness and in their use of medical facilities. Whereas the English-speaking people preferred modern medical science and hospitalization, the Spanish-speaking people were more likely to rely on folk medicine and family care and support.

The traditional concern about health among Jewish

persons, especially as regards their children, can sometimes lead to overconcern and encourage doubts and
anixety. Such concern can also encourage a high standard of infant rearing and caring. This was clearly supported by an early study of infant mortality among im-
migrants to America which showed that although the
Jewish group was foreign born, had just as many children and had an income much lower than that of native
born whites, they had the lowest rate of infant mortality of all the groups studied.

In summary, the following are the types of variables
affecting response to illness:

1. Visibility and recognizability of signs and
   symptoms.
2. The extent to which the symptoms are perceived
   as serious.
3. The extent to which the symptoms disrupt normal functioning.
4. The frequency and persistence of the signs or
   symptoms.
5. The tolerance threshold of the individual.
6. Available information, knowledge, and understanding of the individual.
7. Basic needs that lead to denial.
8. Needs competing with illness responses.
9. Competing interpretations that can be assigned
   to the symptoms.
10. Availability of treatment resources and psycho-
    logical and financial effects of taking action.

The Medical Market Place

As populations demand more medical care, there is
growing concern to provide a minimal level of service
to all and to decrease obvious inadequacies. Thus, there

is a tendency to link existing services to defined population groups, to develop new and economic ways to provide primary care services to the population without too great an emphasis on technology, to integrate services increasingly fragmented by specialization, and to seek ways to improve the output of the delivery system with fixed inputs. Furthermore, because of the high and growing cost of providing health services, the value of increased provision of health care has to be weighed in relation to other social needs and political contingencies. Governments—like people—have limited resources and must make decisions about how to distribute these resources in dealing with competing demands.

From the perception of community health, it is important that services be available to people who need them and who can most benefit from them—and it is essential that the quality of these services be maintained and developed. It must be further recognized that most of the major diseases producing mortality or morbidity are not well understood, and existing efforts, while they may ameliorate suffering and sometimes extend life, are extremely expensive. To name a few examples—hemodialysis and transplantation in end-stage kidney disease, coronary by-pass surgery, radiation therapy for cancer, and the development of a variety of intensive care units.

In order to assess the amount of society's resources that should be devoted to health care there are two general methodologies—planning and the marketplace. The subject of health planning is discussed in another chapter of this book. Here we will be concerned only with the marketplace.

The marketplace model is based on the premise that the consumer is in the best position to determine the value he places on a particular product or service.

Accordingly, this point of view would hold that the marketplace is the best means of determining the amount of health care people want relative to other commodities and services. In response to the argument that some people have too little money to buy health care, advocates would argue that they should be given money to spend in terms of their own priorities and preferences rather than have outsiders determine what they need. On the other hand, from the point of view of many medical care experts, the medical marketplace in the United States does not distribute medical services in a fair or cost-effective manner. Clearly, providing basic medical services to groups in the population that have not had adequate care will probably have an important impact on their health; however, offering more and more services to those already well-provided for is less likely to contribute to better health.

The medical marketplace, as it exists in the United States is a complex mixture of private and public involvement, social regulations, and professional governance. Medical care involves so many exceptions to traditional economic assumptions that application of the marketplace model is dubious.

Obviously, the consumer is faced with many problems in assessing the value of medical care and generally places his confidence and trust in the physician from whom he seeks care and who, he assumes, has the requisite knowledge to make the "right" decision. Furthermore, many patients who are anxious and worried have serious psychologic barriers to receiving and analyzing information about their medical condition.

Related to the problem of the consumer's lack of information is the uncertainty of the marketed product. Recovery from disease is, after all, as unpredictable as its incidence. Moreover, it is not always easy for even the physician to determine which services are discretionary and which mandatory. Although patients can theoretically refuse to agree to physicians' decisions, they usually have no basis for doing so.

The irregular and unexpected character of medical demand has important implications for consumers. Most people assume that the medical sector could respond effectively to any eventuality; they lose sight of the fact that while frequently occurring diseases are usually properly provided for, others are sometimes neglected. Even some common ailment may be neglected under certain circumstances, for example, mental retardation or chronic diseases of old age. Another factor of some importance is that the law of supply and demand does not appear to be operative in the medical marketplace as it is in the purchase of commodities; prices do not appear to be particularly responsive to changing demand. As an example, one need only cite the cost of general surgery in areas having an excess of surgeons. It has been often stated that physicians create their own demand.

REFERENCES

Clairborne, Robert: A penny of prevention—The cure for America's health care system, Sunday Review, Jan. 6, 1979.

Mechanic, David: *Medical Sociology*, 2nd ed., New York, Macmillan Publishing Co., 1978.

Hennes, D. James: The measurement of health, Medical Care Review 29, December, 1972.

Koos, E.: *The Health of Regionsville; What People Thought and Did About It*, New York, Columbia University Press, 1954.

Saunders, L.: *Cultural Differences in Medical Care; The Case of the Spanish-speaking People of the South West*, New York, Russel Sage Foundation, 1954.

Chapter 7

Environmental Factors in Disease Prevention

WATER SUPPLY

In addition to being used for human consumption, water is required for many other purposes; these include its use for agricultural and recreational purposes, for industry, in the disposal of human and industrial wastes, for fire-fighting, and as a medium for transportation. The average daily consumption of water per capita has grown fairly rapidly in the United States and is currently estimated at approximately 230 gallons.

Water has long been known as a source of transmission of disease. Those diseases known to be spread by water may be divided into bacterial, viral and parasitic infections. Among the bacterial diseases are listed cholera, bacillary dysentery, typhoid fever, and leptospirosis. Among the viral infections are included infectious hepatitis and probably poliomyelitis, while among the parasitic infections there are amebiasis and schistosomiasis.

Rapid growth has characterized the development of community water supplies in the United States during this century. In 1900, only 3,200 cities and towns had community water systems, while today some 58,000 public water supply systems serving 15 or more persons are being operated in this country. During this period, death rates from enteric infections, including typhoid and the dysenteries, fell rapidly. The widespread epidemics of disease due to pollution of water supplies which were once common occurrences have been essentially eliminated in those municipalities which have developed public water supplies.

Sources of Water

The sources of our water supply may be divided into three general groups:

1. Rain or snow water
2. Surface water, including rivers, lakes, streams and ponds
3. Ground water, including springs and wells

Rain Water. Rain water would normally be considered to be the most satisfactory source of water in terms of purity; however, it is quite difficult to collect in such a way as to render it reasonably free from pollution in any quantity and is, therefore, not particularly suitable as a direct source of water for any sizeable population group.

Surface Water. The liability of surface water to pollution from waste and from surface wash is very large and, therefore, in general, it is not possible to consider such water safe for drinking without appropriate treatment. The most important sources of pollution are human, industrial and agricultural waste, with particular emphasis on human waste as a possible source of disease.

Ground Water. Water that is taken from springs and

wells is often less polluted than is surface water. However, *springs* are usually shallow and difficult to protect from surface pollution. *Wells* may be shallow or deep. There are five common types of wells, depending upon the way in which they have been developed.

1. Dug wells are usually excavated by hand, are normally relatively shallow, and usually penetrate only a short distance into the water-bearing strata.
2. Bored wells are commonly constructed with earth augers turned either by hand or by power equipment. In suitable overlay, holes from 2 to 30 inches in diameter can be bored to about 100 feet.
3. Driven wells are the simplest and least expensive to construct. The yield of driven wells is usually small to moderate and their depth is limited.
4. Jetted wells are developed by sinking the well point by jetting or washing-in. The well point and pipe are pushed down as material is loosened by the jetting. This type of well is limited in depth and by soil characteristics.
5. Drilled wells are ordinarily developed by percussion or rotary drilling in good water-bearing strata and can be developed to produce a dependable supply and large quantities of water; they may tap water-bearing strata at considerable depths below the surface. These wells constitute the most satisfactory method by which ground waters can be developed.

It is essential to protect wells from surface drainage and surface contamination by ensuring that a watertight seal is provided around the top of the well casing. It is also important to avoid contamination of well water supplies by ensuring that the sewage disposal system is not placed in proximity to the well. It is also very desirable to ensure that the well water supply is placed above the level of the sewage disposal system or privy so that the material from the human waste cannot reach the source of well water.

Treatment

Treatment is designed to remove turbidity, color, taste and odor, as well as to disinfect water. Clarification of water is carried out primarily through filtration and disinfection by chlorination. Its purpose is to prevent the transmission of disease to man.

Filtration. The primary function of filtration is to remove through this process those materials that can be filtered out. In water treatment, coagulation by chemicals, such as alum, is followed by sedimentation for a period of time during which the flocculent particles are allowed to settle. The clarified water is then filtered through a bed of sand and gravel. The filter is cleaned by reversing the flow of water through the filter. Chlorine is usually applied before and after filtration.

Disinfection. The desirable properties for a chemical disinfectant include high germicidal power, stability, solubility, non-toxicity to man and animals, economy, dependability, residual effect, ease of use and measurement, and availability. Compounds of chlorine most satisfactorily comply with the properties of a chemical disinfectant. Chlorine, which is an oxidizing agent, is the commonly used water disinfectant. The amount of chlorine necessary to provide adequate protection must satisfy the chlorine demand of organic and other oxidizable material in the water and provide a residual chlorine concentration which will ensure proper disinfection.

Emergency Disinfection. If required, this can be accomplished by boiling the water for one minute or by adding a few drops of either chlorine bleach or iodine. If chlorine or iodine is used, the water should be allowed to stand for about a half-hour after treatment before it is used. Aerating boiled water will improve its taste.

SEWAGE DISPOSAL

Inasmuch as human wastes constitute the most important source of contamination of water and therefore the production of human disease through this medium, an understanding of methods of waste disposal aimed at ensuring the protection of sources of water is essential. Waste disposal systems may be divided, for our purposes, into two general groups:

1. Individual disposal systems
2. Community disposal systems

Individual Disposal Systems

Privies. The pit privy, still extensively used, particularly in rural areas, constitutes a safe and satisfactory method of waste disposal where water carriage systems of disposal cannot be utilized. However to ensure its safety, the location of the privy, its construction, and its maintenance are all important. The privy should be located a reasonable distance from any source of ground water supply and at a lower elevation than the water source. The bottom of the pit should be some distance above the ground water. The privy should have a self-closing door in order to prevent contamination by flies.

Chemical Toilets. Chemical toilets have been used where it is necessary to have toilet facilities in or near a building, but where running water under pressure is not available, or where soil conditions make subsurface disposal of sewage unsatisfactory. The toilet consists

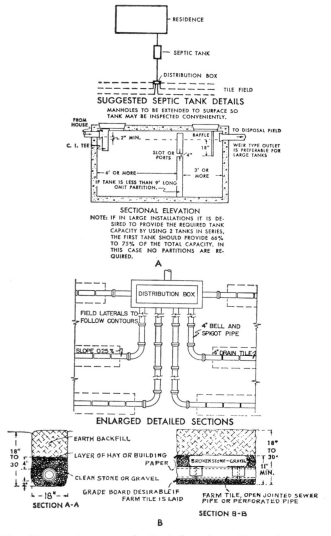

Fig. 17. A, Septic tank. B, Subsurface disposal of septic tank effluent. (Hilleboe and Larimore: *Preventive Medicine*, 2nd Ed., Philadelphia, W. B. Saunders Co.)

merely of a pail located beneath the seat, containing a chemical solution, most commonly sodium hydroxide. This type was once commonly used as home emergency toilets or on boats and mobile homes.

Subsurface Sewage Disposal System

This includes a septic tank which is a water-tight unit, usually made of concrete or steel. The tank normally retains the sewage for approximately 24 hours in order to separate the solids from the liquid waste. The liquid is discharged from the tank and flows into a disposal field which consists of a series of perforated pipes placed in trenches approximately 2 feet deep and 2 feet wide. These pipes are laid in coarse gravel and the liquid effluent seeps into the adjoining soil.

In order for a subsurface disposal system to function properly, it is essential that the soil be capable of absorbing the liquid. Testing in advance to ensure that the effluent will, in fact, continue to be absorbed properly into the soil is essential. The septic tank itself must be cleaned out at regular intervals because of sludge deposits and scum accumulation. It is essential that the subsurface sewage disposal system be located where it will not pollute any water supply from a well or spring. It should be located at a distance from any water supply source and, if possible, at a lower elevation. The location should be determined by a competent public health engineer or sanitarian from the local health department.

Community Disposal Systems

The overall function of a community sewage disposal system is to collect all of the liquid waste from that community, to convey it to a treatment plant, and to provide treatment aimed at removing a sufficient part of the organic, inorganic and bacterial material, so that ultimate disposal of the liquid effluent may be effected without creating a pollutional problem in the receiving water, thus avoiding jeopardy to the health of the public or interference with the propagation of fish and wildlife. The system should also ensure that the effluent being deposited does not interfere with the use of the water course for recreational or other purposes. The system starts at the individual home or office where the waste is deposited into pipes which join into common sewers, which in turn reach to the sewage treatment plant. At the treatment plant, the waste material is channeled through coarse or bar screens which remove some of the larger solids; it is then put through a grit chamber which removes some of the heavy mineral and inorganic material in the waste. The effluent is then channeled into a settling tank in which slow settling of solids can take place. This whole process is called *primary treatment.*

The solid material that has settled out from the sewage is placed in large tanks to digest. After a period of digestion of some 30 to 60 days, depending upon the temperature, it is dehydrated either on rotary filters or on sludge drying beds. This material is commonly known as sludge and often has been used as fertilizer. It should be noted, however, that studies have indicated that even when digested sludge has remained exposed to the atmosphere for many months, it is possible to isolate pathogenic organisms from the material. It is important, therefore, to be sure that care is exercised when sludge is utilized for soil-improvement purposes.

An Imhoff tank is a special kind of primary treatment unit which has a purpose similar to that of a simple primary sedimentation-settling tank, except that the settling solids in the Imhoff tank pass through a slot in

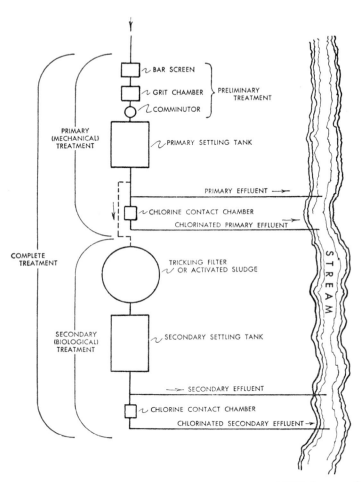

Fig. 18.   Complete treatment processes. (Hilleboe and Larimore: *Preventive Medicine*, 2nd Ed., Philadelphia, W. B. Saunders Co.)

the bottom of the tank to a sludge compartment beneath. The sludge then remains in the digestion compartment until it decomposes.

Primary treatment may be followed by chlorination aimed at producing some degree of disinfection in the effluent. However, primary treatment is usually insufficient even when augmented by chlorination of the effluent to meet the requirements of most systems for water quality criteria for receiving streams.

Secondary treatment includes further treatment of the liquid effluent and is usually accompanied by aerobic biologic methods such as trickling filters or aeration. It adds considerable expense to the treatment process. The function of these processes is essentially to remove a major portion of the dissolved organic matter in the liquid waste which cannot be removed by the process of settling. The effluent from the secondary treatment may also be chlorinated just prior to discharge to the water course. Again, the major purpose of this chlorination process is to destroy pathogenic organisms to the greatest extent possible.

The rapid growth of community sewage disposal systems, in spite of the expense involved, can be gleaned from the fact that in 1900 only some 950 communities had community systems, whereas today there are approximately 17,000 public systems in existence.

WATER POLLUTION

Pollution of our nation's water courses has been a problem of concern to health and conservation agencies for many years. Contributing factors include the discharge of human wastes, either untreated or inadequately treated, the rapid growth of industrial production, with its concomitant discharge of industrial waste into streams and rivers, and run-off from agricultural land. Thus, it can be seen readily that a variety of pollutants are contaminating our waterways. These include not only human and animal sewage, but a great variety of chemicals, including those used as detergents, pesticides and fertilizers, as well as trash, etc., and a variety of organic matter. More recently, still another contaminant has been introduced, i.e., radioactivity.

These various pollutants have had a substantial adverse effect on the "quality" of these rivers and streams. Clearly, they preclude or make very difficult and expensive the use of such water as a source of drinking water, not only because of the introduction of harmful bacteria and chemical substances, but because of the development of objectionable taste and odor in the affected water. In addition, they have, on many occasions, been responsible for killing fish, and they certainly have prevented these waters from being used for recreational purposes.

While laws have been established in many states aimed at the control of water pollution, such laws have proved difficult to enforce, primarily because of the great expense involved in providing adequate treatment of both human and industrial waste. Nevertheless, the implementation of this type of control program is essential if our waterways are to be reclaimed for appropriate public uses.

SWIMMING POOLS

Because of the possibility of communicable diseases, such as eye, ear, nose and throat infections, as well as some fungal infections of the skin being transmitted through bathing facilities, considerable attention is usually placed on the sanitation of these facilities by the official public health agency.

Usually, the health agency is called upon to review

the plans for the construction of the pool and its environs. In this way a number of public health engineering hazards can be avoided. Such a procedure may also serve to prevent considerable expense on the part of the owner who may have to correct deficiencies after the facilities have been constructed.

It is essential that filtered water be continually recirculated and adequately chlorinated and that there be an adequate mechanism for the prevention of back flow. There should be no connection between the water supply or swimming pool drain and the sewage disposal system. Appropriate facilities should be designed to ensure the provision of safety precautions for swimmers, not only in the pool but also in its environs.

During operation of the pool, the chlorine residual should be continually checked to be sure that it does not fall below acceptable standards. Every effort should be made to maintain cleanliness in the dressing room and bathhouse areas. Persons having communicable diseases, or eye or ear infections, should be excluded from using the pool to the extent that this is feasible. Adequate lifesaving equipment and safety devices should be readily available, and lifeguards should be on continuous duty. First aid kits should be available and accessible at all times.

MILK

Milk has long been known to be an important carrier of human disease. Among the diseases transmissible through milk are typhoid, dysentery, tuberculosis, streptococcal infections, brucellosis, salmonella infections, diphtheria, infectious hepatitis, poliomyelitis and Q fever. Pasteurization has been extremely effective in preventing many of the wide-spread milk-borne outbreaks that previously prevailed. Such outbreaks still occur in areas where protection of the milk supply from contamination is not adequate. Milk may be contaminated by direct contact with animals or persons, through dirty utensils or polluted wash water, or by intermediate agents, such as flies or rats. Most of the diseases spread by fluid milk can also be transmitted by milk products.

Milk Sanitation

Milk serves as an excellent culture medium for bacteria. A safe and sanitary supply of milk is assured by protection at three levels:

1. Production
2. Processing
3. Distribution

Production. Bacteria present in milk originate from the animal, the milk handlers, and the environment in which milking is carried out. The bacterial count of raw milk is the best indication of the sanitary conditions under which milk is produced and handled. The bacterial content depends upon the cleanliness and health of the animal and the milkers and on the cleanliness of the milking utensils as well as on the rate of cooking and length of time and temperature at which the raw milk is stored. Protection of the cows, care in the use of insecticides and fly control are also important. Methods of transportation must be carefully controlled.

Processing. The processing of milk and milk products has as its major objectives:

1. Destruction of pathogenic organisms
2. Improvement of the keeping quality without important loss of flavor or nutritive properties
3. Removal of tastes and odors

4. Fortification, for example, with vitamins
5. Homogenization

The organisms are destroyed by the process of heat treatment, commonly known as pasteurization. The pasteurization process includes heating, holding and rapid cooling. The milk is either heated to a temperature of 145° F and kept at that temperature at least 30 minutes, or the high temperature-short time method is used in which the milk is heated to at least 161° F and held at this temperature for at least 15 seconds. The milk is then rapidly cooled to 45° F or below, bottled, and maintained at this temperature until it is ready for marketing. This method, if properly carried out, is effective in destroying pathogenic bacteria.

The *phosphatase test* is a useful laboratory test designed to deterimne whether or not the milk has been properly pasteurized. When milk is properly pasteurized, the phosphatase is essentially destroyed. In cases of under-pasteurization, the presence of phosphatase will be revealed.

Distribution. In the delivery, storage and handling of milk until it reaches the consumer, it is essential that the milk be maintained at refrigeration temperatures, 45° F or less, at all times. Original containers of milk should not be opened nor should any of the contents be removed before the product reaches the consumer.

FOOD

Diseases which may be transmitted by food are as follows: tapeworm infestations, trichinosis, amebic and bacillary dysentery, cholera, typhoid, tularemia, tuberculosis, infectious hepatitis, and "food poisoning." From this list, it is evident that the control of food infection is an important public health measure.

Food-borne Illness (Food Poisoning)

What we commonly call "food poisoning" is characterized by acute onset of nausea, vomiting, diarrhea, abdominal cramps, and fever of varying degree. Food poisoning may be divided into three general groups: toxic, bacterial, and chemical.

Toxic Food Poisoning. There are two major categories of food poisoning produced by bacterial toxins. By far the most common of these is *staphylococcal food poisoning*. This disease is characterized by acute symptoms which usually occur in 2 to 4 hours after ingestion of contaminated food. The patient usually feels much better after 24 hours. Outbreaks of staphylococcal food poisoning in the United States are common and are usually due to contamination of food from infections existing on the body of the food handler, typically boils on the hands or other body surfaces. The staphylococcus produces enterotoxin, which is the factor involved in producing the symptoms. The most common kinds of foods implicated in staphylococcal food poisoning are milk and milk products and custard or cream-filled pastries; meat has also been incriminated in a number of outbreaks.

Prevention of staphylococcal food poisoning involves education of food handlers, restriction of workers from handling food if they have obvious sores on the hands or other exposed surfaces, and ensuring that food is maintained hot (above 140° F) or under refrigeration (below 45° F) and not left to stand at atmospheric temperatures for a long time.

Botulism occurs much less frequently than does staphylococcal poisoning, but is a highly fatal food intoxication produced as the result of ingestion of food in which the toxin of *Clostridium botulinum* has been produced. The incubation period is usually from 12 to 36 hours and is followed by muscular weakness and visual disturbance. Diplopia usually occurs, often accompanied by vertigo. There is difficulty in talking and swallowing, followed by incoordination, respiratory paralysis and death. Gastroenteric symptoms are quite variable and may be minor. Botulism is usually produced as the result of ingestion of infected canned vegetables and fruits. *Clostridium botulinum* normally requires anaerobic conditions to survive and multiply. These conditions may, of course, be produced in canned vegetables, particularly in those canned at home. Lightly smoked fish, vacuum sealed in plastic wrap, has also been implicated. There is a specific antitoxin available for use in the treatment of botulism. However, once the disease occurs, the mortality rate is high. Prevention is therefore all important and consists of proper education of householders in safe methods of home canning.

Bacterial Food Poisoning. Bacterial food poisoning is commonly due to a member of the genus of microorganisms known as Salmonella; the disease is called salmonellosis. Salmonellosis is characterized by an incubation period of approximately 12 hours' duration. It is quite similar in character to staphylococcal food poisoning, although it may be somewhat more severe. and recovery usually takes a little longer, approximately 48 hours. Salmonellosis is produced as the result of infection of food by human carriers or by infection already being present in the food at the time it is prepared. The most commonly infected foods are fowl and eggs. Prevention of salmonellosis involves education of food handlers in methods of cooking and refrigerating food. Cooking at approximately 165° F for at least 2 minutes will destroy salmonellae.

It should also be pointed out that there are other organisms undoubtedly capable of producing bacterial food poisoning. However, it has been difficult to prove conclusively that these other organisms have been actually responsible. Among those incriminated are *Streptococcus faecalis*, *Clostridium welchii* and *Bacillus cereus*. There is, however, one important group or organisms that should be mentioned as important etiologic agents. These are the dysentery bacilli (Shigella). They produce a more severe type of illness, sometimes fatal. Of the dysenteries, *Shigella sonnei* is quite common in some countries.

Chemical Food Poisoning. This occurs, usually, as the result of accidental contamination of food by insecticides, cleaning materials or metals. Examples include poisoning from cyanide in silver polishes and from sodium fluoride and arsenate used in insecticides. Cadmium-plating and other metal coatings on containers or utensils have also been implicated. The illness is characterized by acute onset approximately one-half hour after eating, with prominent nausea and vomiting. Prevention clearly involves the use of care in storage and utilization of insecticides, polishes and other materials in which harmful chemicals may be found.

A number of poisonous plants occasionally produce food poisoning; among the most common of these is the mushroom. Symptoms of mushroom poisoning usually appear soon after eating (in 15 to 30 minutes). Liver damage and death may occur if sufficient mushroom toxin has been ingested. There is no effective treatment other than gastric lavage, together with the use of atropine, a specific antidote to the mushroom toxin (muscarine). Another poisoning which is not uncommon is mussel poisoning; this has occurred particularly in the San Francisco and Bay of Fundy areas.

This, again, is the result of a toxin present in the mussels. It is characterized by early onset of illness, followed by muscle weakness and respiratory paralysis. Aside from gastric lavage there is little else that can be done, although in cases in which respiratory distress occurs, oxygen may be administered.

Food Sanitation

Health departments throughout the country spend a good deal of time in supervising and inspecting restaurants and other food establishments. The primary objective of this program is, of course, to prevent the spread of illness through the medium of food. The success of such a program depends upon several factors.

Food Handler Education. Those engaged in the preparation and handling of foods must fully understand the methods by which food may serve to spread disease and the precautions that need to be taken in order to prevent such diseases from occurring or spreading. Classes for food handlers, therefore, are of great value in providing instruction to those employed in the industry. The proper cleaning and handling of equipment and food, accompanied by cleanliness on the part of the individual food handler, will play a key role in the prevention of food-borne disease. Any food handler who has lesions on his hands or other exposed parts of the body should not participate in food handling until the lesion has been cleared up. A food handler who has recently had a bout of diarrhea should certainly have stool specimens taken to ensure that he is not carrying pathogenic bacteria which can be transmitted through food. Proper hand-washing and personal hygiene are essential barriers against contamination of food.

Conditions in the Food Establishment. Equipment

and the interior of the food establishment itself need to be of the types which can be easily cleaned. Insect and rodent control programs are important in food preparation areas. Care should be taken in the storage of insecticides, cleaning compounds and other non-food items so as to avoid the accidental contamination of food by these products. Covering of food to prevent contamination is also important. Water-proof containers with tight-fitting covers should be used in storing garbage at the food establishment. Today in many, if not most, establishments, garbage grinders have been installed.

Temperature Control. Most bacteria do not grow well in cool temperatures and are commonly killed by heating. Adequate refrigeration or cooking of foods is therefore extremely important as a method of preventing food-borne disease.

Proper Preparation of Food. Cooking is an essential procedure in killing pathogenic bacteria. Most bacteria capable of causing disease are readily destroyed by thorough cooking. Trichinosis is one disease which could be eliminated if garbage that is fed to hogs were thoroughly cooked. Proper dishwashing is important as a means of removing scraps in which bacteria can grow. Modern dishwashers, when properly operated, are effective in ensuring that dishes are properly sanitized and cleaned.

In the routine inspection program carried on by health departments, swabbing of dishes, utensils and working surfaces followed by laboratory testing is often carried out to determine the bacterial count. This is a useful device employed as a control mechanism in the inspection program.

INSECTS AND RODENTS

Among the diseases spread by insect vectors or rodents are typhus, plague, Rocky Mountain spotted fever, tularemia, rickettsialpox, typhoid, bacillary and amebic dysentery, trypanosomiasis, leishmaniasis, malaria, yellow fever, filariasis and encephalitis. While it is true that many of these diseases are more or less confined to countries outside of the United States, several do occur here. The control of insects and rodents is therefore of considerable importance. Control of insect vectors is accomplished by a combination of five procedures:

1. Chemical control
2. Elimination of breeding sites
3. The control of infected animals which may carry the insect vectors
4. The use of insect repellants for exposed persons
5. The protection of human beings by immunization or by chemoprophylaxis

It has been said that in the major cities of the United States the rat population may be measured by assuming that there is roughly one rat for each human resident in the city. The basis of rodent control consists of:

1. Reduction of rat harborage by rat-proofing buildings, and other controls.
2. Making food supply unavailable by proper disposal of garbage.
3. Eradication by the use of rodenticides and by trapping and gassing.

HOUSING

Winslow has said, "The filth epidemics of the 19th century have been conquered in civilized and relatively prosperous lands like ours. We can now think in terms of health rather than in terms of disease; and, from this standpoint, such problems as nutrition and housing come to the forefront. The slum of today is no longer the hot-bed of cholera and typhus fever as it was 75 years ago. It remains, however, one of the major obstacles to that physical and emotional and social vigor and efficiency and satisfaction which we conceive as the health objective of the future."

Although many attempts have been made to establish a clear relationship between health and housing, conclusive evidence has so far not been forthcoming; this is primarily because of the fact that individuals who live under poor housing conditions are usually those of low socioeconomic status and, as such, are liable to a higher incidence of disease. In spite of the difficulties involved in proving conclusively that a relationship exists, it is generally accepted that health agencies have an important role to play in improving levels of housing and general housing conditions. Certainly, it is well known that large numbers of dwellings in the United States are over-crowded, and lack hot and cold running water or decent toilet facilities. Many have no bathtub or shower.

Improvement of housing conditions is aimed at:

1. Planning for the future development of our communities
2. The reduction of health and accident hazards
3. The elimination of grossly deteriorated housing
4. Rehabilitation of substandard housing
5. Control of new construction and remodeling

Numerous factors usually are given consideration. Each dwelling unit requires:

1. A sufficient number of rooms, floor area and volume of space to satisfy human requirements for health and family life
2. A potable water supply provided by proper sanitary plumbing

3. A safe and sanitary method of sewage disposal and removal of garbage and refuse
4. Proper washing and bathing facilities
5. Necessary facilities for cooking, eating and food storage
6. Protection against heat, cold and dampness
7. Adequate ventilation
8. Adequate illumination

Most communities have a building or housing code which makes reference to these and other factors; other requirements may be applicable, including such items as freedom from insect and rodent infestation, proper structural maintenance, means of egress, adequate sleeping facilities, etc. Protection against accidents is particularly important in considering the hygiene of housing. This protection should include the provision of adequate facilities for escape in case of fire, protection against danger of electrical shocks, protection against traffic hazards in the neighborhood where the home is located.

PESTICIDES

Today, pesticides are used in vast quantities in agriculture, in industry, in the home and on the farm. Some of these find their way into the food, milk and water that human beings consume. The quantities of pesticides found in our food, milk, and other beverages vary considerably. While we are well aware of the danger of these substances when they are ingested in large quantities, data are not available which indicate clearly to what extent, if any, there is danger to humans from ingesting pesticides in small quantities over a long time. Nevertheless, it would appear clear that steps must be taken to reduce the pesticide content of our food, milk and water. However, this is not simple. Once an animal has ingested pesticide in its feed, it may take many months before it will excrete or detoxify all of the chemical.

Since DDT was first commercially introduced in 1945, the quantity of pesticide chemicals used in this country has increased tremendously. Furthermore, the use of these chemicals is likely to continue to increase in the future. Large numbers of different chemicals are now employed. Most of these are stable, so that their toxic effects persist for long periods after the chemicals are first applied. Almost all pesticides are potentially harmful to human health. Factors that must be considered in relation to this danger include the toxicity of the chemical, the dose applied, the ability of the chemical to persist in toxic form, and the exact amounts and length of time to which a population is exposed. Currently available data on the toxicity of pesticides are not adequate to evaluate with certainty their safety or the degree of health hazards involved in their use. However, a considerable number of pesticide-related outbreaks have been reported among agricultural workers. Most of these have involved exposure to organophosphates; the symptoms have generally been relatively mild.

GARBAGE AND REFUSE

The amount of garbage and refuse that must be collected and disposed of amounts to approximately half-a-ton per person per year. Much garbage is now disposed of in home and industrial garbage grinders; the material eventually finds its way into the sewers and is disposed of with human waste material. However, vast quantities of trash and garbage remain for collection and disposal. Before collection, refuse should be stored in tight-fitting containers to avoid spillage and exposure to rodents and flies. Collections are usually made once or twice a week.

Many communities still dispose of garbage and refuse in open dumps which become the breeding ground for rodents and flies, as well as being unsightly. There are several modern methods of disposal. However, the one most applicable depends on the particular situation obtaining in the area concerned.

The Sanitary Land-fill

This method of disposal is particularly useful where land is readily available at not too great a distance from the area to be served. If the land is low-lying, it is often possible to reclaim it for possible use as a recreational area after a few years of sanitary land-fill operations. Briefly, in sanitary land-fill, the garbage and refuse is disposed of in previously-dug trenches and is then covered with earth.

Incineration

This is another popular method for disposal of garbage and refuse. Incinerators, however, tend to be fairly expensive to build and maintain. Furthermore, construction should avoid creating an air pollution problem. It should also be borne in mind that, even after incineration, approximately a third of the material remains as ash to be disposed of in some other way.

Dumping at Sea

This is a method often employed by seacoast towns. It tends to be a fairly inexpensive method, but some of the material often finds its way back to the shore, and may also interfere with fishing activities.

AIR POLLUTION

The problem of air pollution has engaged the attention of health agencies only during recent years. Industry has for many years discharged its waste materials into the air without regard to its possible effect on human beings. Homes, public buildings, trains, buses, oil refineries and automobiles all contribute to the general contamination of the air.

Interest in the problem of air pollution was aroused in the United States in October 1948, when an episode occurred in Donora, Pennsylvania, which resulted in illness of more than a third of the population and death of 18 persons.

Characteristics of Atmospheric Contamination

The average person views air pollution as a problem primarily involving direct nuisances, such as the soot or fly ash drifting down from the neighborhood laundry or home heating unit or the odors emitted from the neighboring kitchen exhaust fan. The fact of the matter is, however, that the real problem is not so simple or precise. In its broad perspective, the air pollution problem includes all the contributing sources from the small home heating unit to the colossal steel manufacturing plants and power generating plants of our thriving and ever-growing world economy. The sum total of this aerial garbage mixed into the thin layer of atmosphere that surrounds us has only to become stagnant for short periods before the concentration of pollutants builds up to levels which cause huge economic losses as a result of soiling and dirtying of our homes, offices and buildings, household goods and clothing; corrosion of metals and the erosion of our buildings; damage to protective coatings such as paints and destruction of agricultural crops, trees, shrubbery, and damage to livestock. Of far more importance, it causes discomfort and, on occasion, illness and even death to human beings, as indicated in the Donora episode cited above.

The air pollution problem is well exemplified by the Los Angeles smog which commonly produces irritation of the eyes and damage to plants. Much of this is due to the absence of wind and to the incomplete combustion of gasoline by the many thousands of automobiles in the Los Angeles area, although air pollution from industry and from homes contributes to the total atmospheric pollution.

Following the Donora incident and others, such as that which occurred in London in December 1952, resulting in 4,000 deaths in excess of normal figures, it became increasingly clear that air pollution has an effect upon human health and can cause acute illness and death. Much more difficult to document are the long-term effects of exposure to low concentrations of air pollutants which may result in gradual deterioration of health, chronic disease, and perhaps premature death. However, an impressive body of circumstantial evidence is accumulating which tends to link air pollution with increased mortality from cardiorespiratory disease, increased susceptibility to disease, and interference with normal respiratory functions. This evidence comes from three main types of investigation:

1. Statistical studies of past morbidity and mortality correlated with geographic location and other factors associated with air pollution
2. Epidemiologic studies of morbidity and respiratory functions as related to variations in air pollution
3. Laboratory studies of response by animals and by humans, in some cases, to exposure to various pollutants, singularly or in combination

A few examples of results from these studies are of interest. Death rates from cardiorespiratory diseases in the United States are greater in urban than in rural areas and, in general, increase with city size. Within the past few years, this urban-rural difference has also shown up in the mortality of infants. Variations within cities have also been demonstrated. In one large midwestern city, cardiorespiratory death rates in census tracts within one mile of a large primary metal manufacturing district exceeded by sevenfold the rates in other areas matched for socioeconomic conditions but located two to three times as far away.

Although the examples cited provide circumstantial evidence only and cannot be taken as proving a cause-and-effect relationship between air pollution and chronic effects upon health, mounting information clearly indicates that there is strong need to control air pollution.

There are three major factors involved in the production of air pollution. In addition to the methods by which contamination is produced and the factor of population density which is related thereto, the other important factors are weather and terrain. Most notable air pollution incidents have occurred in lowland valleys or river plains during periods of high humidity and temperature inversion. Temperature inversion is produced when warm air prevents the normal upward displacement of air and its contaminants. This results in a retention of these contaminants and their accumulation in the lower stratum. Thus, the Los Angeles smog results not only from the combustion products of thousands of automobiles, but also from the topographic features of the area, which lead to the accumulation of a large air pocket over the city, especially in summer and early fall when temperature inversions are likely to occur.

Relationship between Air Pollution and Human Disease

The Donora and London incidents previously cited, along with several others that have occurred in past years, have clearly revealed a close relationship between episodes of air pollution and the development of acute sickness and the occurrence, even, of death. Most commonly, as in the Los Angeles smog, air pollution produces irritation of the eyes. There is, of course, little question of the relationship between the development of hay fever and air pollution; it is well known that hay fever results from various plant allergens suspended in the air. Data developed in Great Britain would also appear to indicate a relationship between air pollution and a variety of chronic pulmonary diseases, including bronchitis and emphysema. Questions have been raised concerning the possible relationship of air pollution over long periods of time with the development of lung cancer; however, the evidence is far from conclusive.

Another question which should be discussed concerns the adverse effect of air pollution on a population with pre-existing pulmonary or cardiac disease. The Donora incident has produced rather conclusive evidence that, in fact, a definite deleterious effect exists in such instances.

Control Measures

The Environmental Protection Agency has recently attempted to summarize what is known and what is unknown about the health effects of air pollution. It states "The adverse health effects of air pollution are widespread and costly even though they cannot be measured precisely and recorded in a ledger. Sickness means increased costs for medical care, hospitalization, and drugs. Time lost by wage earners is a debit to the persons involved and to the national economy.

"The National Lung Association, after surveying 23 studies made in a 10-year period by government, industry and university scientists and economists, concluded that a reasonable estimate of the health cost of polluted air in the United States is more than $10 billion a year."

It capsulizes scientific studies by indicating that air pollution is related to human sickness and sometimes to premature death. People of both sexes and ages can be affected but the danger is greatest for the very old and the very young and for people already sick with certain chronic ailments such as diseases of the respiratory system and of the heart and blood vessels, cancer, especially of the lungs, and skin diseases, allergies and eye irritation.

Obviously, the complete elimination of air pollution does not appear feasible, so that control measures need primarily to be aimed at reducing the extent to which the problem exists. The essential steps needed for a control program are:

1. A survey aimed at determining the sources and types of air pollution, followed by necessary steps aimed at the reduction of these emissions by appropriate legislation and enforcement programs
2. Study and regulation of industrial plant design in order to reduce the extent of atmospheric pollution
3. Appropriate steps, legislative and other, aimed at the reduction of combustion products in automobile engines
4. A continuous air monitoring program aimed at maintaining surveillance over air quality

5. A public health educational program aimed at informing the public of the possible hazards of air pollution and methods of reduction of this hazard

IONIZING RADIATION

As a result of the increasing use of radiation in industry and medicine in recent years, as well as of the exposure of our population to considerable amounts of radioactivity from the testing of nuclear weapons, the protection of the public against ionizing radiation has become one of our most important public health problems. Ionizing radiation may be produced by certain high energy instruments or by radioactive materials. Radioactive materials may emit alpha, beta or gamma rays. Alpha rays are strongly ionizing, but their penetrating power is so low that they cannot penetrate the skin; beta rays are more penetrating but gamma rays, like x rays, are very penetrating.

Effects on Human Health

Genetic Effects. Genetic effects are produced by irradiation of the reproductive organs and are marked by the appearance of mutations in succeeding generations. This is important because an injury that is not readily apparent to an existing generation may be conveyed to unborn generations. Furthermore, the specific effects appear to be irreversible, so that exposure to small doses of radiation is cumulative.

Other Effects. There is little question that repeated small doses of radiation over a period of time can lead to the development of leukemia. There is more question as to the possibility of development of other cancerous conditions. There appears to be every indication that ionizing radiation to which an individual is exposed does produce some shortening of the life span, the extent of life shortening being directly proportional to the amount of dose; this effect also is cumulative.

The effect of an acute large dose of radiation upon the individual is dramatic. Depending upon the magnitude, the individual may develop, within a few hours, loss of appetite, nausea, vomiting and prostration; if diarrhea occurs during this stage, it indicates that the individual has received a serious and possibly fatal dose; evidence of involvement of the central nervous system also carries a serious prognosis. Following these early symptoms, which may last for approximately 2 days, there is usually a period of 2 to 3 weeks during which the individual is asymptomatic. After the 2 to 3 week interval, there is another period of illness in which the patient may have fever, diarrhea, purpura, central nervous system disorders, epilation and profound weakness. He may succumb to infection, and treatment therefore may include the judicious use of antibiotics.

Development of Radiation Standards

The National Council on Radiation Protection and Measurements has been established to make recommendations concerning safe operating practice in this field. One of the important recommendations of the Council concerns what is known as the maximum permissible dose, MPD. The International Council on Radiation Protection and Measurements has defined the maximum permissible dose* as ". . . . that dose, accumulated over a long period of time or resulting from a single exposure, which, in the light of present knowledge, carries a negligible probability of severe

---

*Recommendations of the ICRP, Publication No. 1, Paragraphs 30 and 31 (London, Pergamon Press, Inc., 1959).

somatic or genetic injuries; furthermore, it is such a dose that any effects that ensue more frequently are limited to those of a minor nature that would not be considered unacceptable by the exposed individual and by the competent medical authorities.

"Any severe somatic injuries (e.g. leukemia) that might result from exposure of individuals to the permissible dose would be limited to an exceedingly small fraction of the exposed group; effects such as shortening of life span which might be expected to occur more frequently, would be very slight and would likely be hidden by normal biological variations. The permissible doses can therefore be expected to produce effects that could be detectable only by statistical methods applied to large groups."

It should be emphasized that it has proven extremely difficult to make recommendations on this subject because there is no threshold dose of radiation below which biologic damage may be avoided. In other words, any dose may be harmful. Therefore, it is always necessary to balance the human risk against the possible benefits accruing from the radiation exposure. Recommendations, therefore, involve difficult judgmental factors, are open to considerable difference of opinion, and are rendered more difficult because effects of radiation are cumulative.

Major Sources of Radiation Exposure

Medical and Dental X Rays. Exposure to these x rays may be divided into two general types: (a) problems created by the use of unsafe x-ray equipment, and (b) problems caused by the careless use of x-ray equipment by persons who have received inadequate training in its use. More than 90% of the man-made ionizing radiation reaching the United States population comes from diagnostic x-ray procedures. In this connection, concomitant with the reduction in tuberculosis, much of the mass chest x-ray screening that was, until recently, in wide use, has now been abandoned in favor of selective tuberculin testing programs.

Clearly, the control of the first problem involves the removal of unsafe equipment or changes in equipment in order to render it safe for use. Control of the second problem involves health education; adequate training must be provided for those who are to use x-ray equipment. There are well-established protection standards for the guidance of manufacturers and users of radiation-producing equipment. These standards have been promulgated as regulations in some local and state jurisdictions. The professional societies and the health agencies may join forces to encourage voluntary cooperation with national protection criteria such as the recommendations of the National Council on Radiation Protection and Measurements. These recommendations are published by the National Bureau of Standards in the form of small handbooks and are available from the Government Printing Office, Washington, D.C., 20401.

Radioactive Isotopes. There are two general classes of radioactive materials—natural and artificially produced—but the properties of each type and the principles of protection from excessive exposure are quite similar. In general, appropriate shielding should be used, and general care must be taken in the time of exposure and the distance at which the individual is exposed. As in the case of x-ray equipment, there are well-established production standards to guide users of radioactive isotopes. In the case of artificially produced materials, most are under the regulatory control of either the United States Atomic Energy Commission or a state or local regulatory agency whose regulations constitute the protection standards. Also the Government Printing Office has handbooks containing the recommendations of the National Council on Radiation Protection and Measurements concerning these sources of radiation.

Radioactive Fallout. Preventive measures which are required in order to control problems related to radioactive fallout thus far have been confined to questions concerning the contamination of the milk supply. Radio-iodine is produced in fairly large amounts during the detonation of nuclear weapons. Depending upon the characteristics of the explosion and the prevailing weather conditions, radioactive iodine may find its way into the milk supply. Most foods other than milk require a considerable time for processing before consumption. The delay may permit the radioactivity to disappear gradually through decay of the radioactive atoms. On the other hand, because of the short time required for processing of milk, it could contain a considerable amount of radio-iodine by the time it is ready for consumption. During the previous periods of atmospheric nuclear testing, only two localities in the nation initiated control measures to minimize exposure to radio-iodine. Control measures, if required, include:

1. Feeding of dairy cows with feeds that have been stored long enough for the radioactivity to decay or with uncontaminated feeds

2. Recommending that young children and pregnant women be placed on evaporated or powdered milk; refrigerated milk, frozen milk, or canned milk which has been stored long enough to reduce the amount of radioactive iodine may also be used

The decision for taking such control measures should be made only after careful evaluation of the problem and is primarily a responsibility of the health agencies of the affected jurisdictions.

Community Radiation Control

The control of radiation as a community responsibility involves a survey of the community to determine where radioactive isotopes are located, and the location and type of x-ray equipment and other radiation-producing devices. This determination of sources of ionizing radiation must be followed by control measures to ensure that they are made as safe as possible. The survey should also be followed by steps to ensure that necessary procedures are effected if an accident occurs with a radioisotope which causes considerable amounts of ionizing radiation to be released into the environment. It is also essential for the community health agency to know when new installations are being established and to maintain surveillance over them. Study of the extent of radioactive material in the food, milk, and water supply followed by appropriate control measures, when necessary, is another important community activity. Medical centers should be encouraged to develop radiation safety programs and to provide for proper transportation, storage and disposal of radioisotopes.

In March 1979, an explosion occurred in the nuclear power plant at Three Mile Island near Harrisburg, Pennsylvania. The resulting national publicity, together with the steps taken to evacuate the immediate area surrounding the plant and to bring conditions at the plant under control afford a recent example of the importance of maintaining continuing surveillance over all sources of radiation.

REFERENCES

Air Pollution and Your Health, Environmental Protection Agency, Washington, D.C., March 1979.

Committee on the Hygiene of Housing: *Basic Principles of Healthful Housing*, New York, American Public Health Association, 1939.

Dach, G. M.: *Food Poisoning*, Revised Ed., Chicago, University of Chicago Press, 1956.

Fair, G. M., *et al.*: *Elements of Water Supply and Waste Water Disposal*, 2nd Ed., New York, John Wiley and Sons, 1971.

Hanlon, J. J.: *Principles of Public Health Administration*, 5th Ed., St. Louis, C. V. Mosby Co., Inc., 1969.

Hilleboe, H. E., and Larimore, G. W.: *Preventive Medicine*, 2nd Ed., Philadelphia, W. B. Saunders Co., 1965.

Hull, T. G.: *Diseases Transmitted from Animals to Man*, 5th Ed., Springfield, Charles C Thomas, 1963.

James, M. T., and Harwood, R. F. (Eds.): *Herms' Medical Entomology*, 6th Ed., New York, The Macmillan Co., 1969.

Magill, P. L., Holden, F. R., and Ackley, C.: *Air Pollution Handbook*, New York, McGraw-Hill Book Co., Inc., 1956.

Moore, E. W., and Fair, G. M.: Water Supply and Waste Disposal, in *Preventive Medicine and Public Health*, 10th Ed., Sartwell, Maxcy and Rosenau, (Eds.): New York, Appleton-Century-Crofts, Inc., 1973.

National Research Council, National Academy of Sciences; The Biological Effects of Atomic Radiation, Summary Reports, Washington, D.C., 1960.

Purdom, R. W.: *Environmental Health*, New York, Academic Press, 1971.

Steel, E. W.: *Water Supply and Sewerage*, 4th Ed., New York, McGraw-Hill Book Co., Inc., 1960.

United States Public Health Service, Division of Radiological Health: *Radiological Health Handbook*, PB 121784 R, Revised Ed., Washington, D.C., 1960.

Weisburd, M. I.: Physicians' guide to air pollution, J.A.M.A. *186*:605, 1963.

World Health Organization: *Milk Hygiene,* New York, Columbia University Press, International Document Service, 1962.

Chapter 8

Maternal and Child Health

Extent of the Problem

Primarily as a result of the great population changes which have occurred, and are still continuing, in and around our great cities, a high percentage of all women and children in these central cities receive prenatal and pediatric care from local health department clinics. The movement of the more affluent members of society to the suburbs and their replacement in the cities by poorer population groups have resulted in local city governments becoming increasingly responsible for providing health services to a growing percentage of the population. In the case of New York City, for example, approximately a third of the infants receive their health supervision from health department well-baby clinics; in some districts this percentage is much higher. In the District of Columbia, a third of all resident births occur at the city's public hospital. This increasing load of tax-supported care is given at public facilities, producing conditions of great overcrowding at many of these and severely taxing their resources. It is difficult in these circumstances to provide high quality care. While the public hospital is overloaded with maternity patients, voluntary hospitals in the city may have only 60 to 70% occupancy in their obstetric departments. About half of all women who have babies at the District of Columbia public hospital have had little or no prenatal care. The prematurity rate is approximately 16%, or more than twice the national rate.

At the Grace-New Haven Community Hospital, it was found that at the hospital emergency room: (1) 43% of the families used this facility as their only source of medical care; (2) 47% of the patients were black, even though blacks represent approximately 6% of New Haven's population; (3) only 20% of the patients were considered to be medical emergencies.

Great progress has been made in the past half century in saving lives of expectant mothers and their infants. Over this period, maternal mortality has declined some 95%, while infant mortality has been reduced by approximately 75%. Many factors have been responsible for this. The general standard of living has risen, nutritional and hygienic standards have improved, and conditions in hospitals have altered radically, while technologic advances in the field of medicine have been great. At the same time, progress in the public health field has also been an important contributing factor, especially in the provision of prenatal care.

In spite of this progress, however, there remains a need for continued efforts to further reduce unnecessary maternal and infant deaths. Beyond this, there is great need to improve the health of expectant mothers and their infants, to exercise preventive techniques, and to reduce the effect of handicapping conditions.

Several studies have demonstrated that the infant and maternal mortality rates vary according to a number of population characteristics. It has been clearly

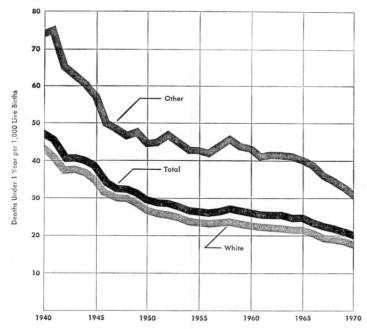

Fig. 19. Infant mortality trends: 1940-1970. (Source of Data: Maternal and Child Health Project, George Washington University.)

established, for example, that these mortality rates vary inversely with socioeconomic status. Genetic, biologic, environmental, social, cultural and economic factors all play important roles in determining these differences. The rate of prematurity is closely related to socioeconomic status. In the District of Columbia, prematurity occurs more than twice as often among black as among white patients.

MATERNAL HEALTH

Maternal Mortality

While it is true that maternal mortality rates have fallen in the United States to little more than 1 per 10,000 live births, problems still exist. For example, it should be noted that the rate is about three times as high in black as in white mothers. Many of the deaths accounting for this difference occur among women delivered outside of hospitals who receive little, if any, medical care during pregnancy. Maternal mortality is also higher in older women. For example, in women 45 years and over the maternal mortality rate is about 12 per 10,000 live births. This appears to be due primarily to complicating diseases.

Some 90% of all maternal deaths result from hemorrhage, infection and toxemia, and many of these still appear to be preventable.

Maternal Health Services

The emphasis in maternal health services, of course, must be on providing adequate prenatal care. This should begin early in pregnancy with monthly visits to the physician, and weekly visits for a month or so prior to the expected delivery date. A complete physical examination at the first visit is required to uncover any medical conditions which need treatment or special handling, as well as to determine the pelvic measurements and condition of the cervix. Blood hemoglobin and grouping (including Rh), serologic tests for syphilis and urinalysis are all essential elements of the examination; a chest x ray should also be taken.

During subsequent visits, the patient should be weighed, her blood pressure should be determined and urinalysis should be performed routinely. Special at-

SECTION 1—GENERAL MORTALITY

Maternal Mortality Rates by Color:
Birth-Registration States or United States, 1915–76

[Prior to 1933, data are for birth-registration States only. Rates per 100,000 live births in specified group. Deaths are classified according to the International Classification of Diseases in use at the time]

Year	Total	White	All other	Year	Total	White	All other
1976	12.3	9.0	26.5	1954	52.4	37.2	143.8
1974[1]	14.6	10.0	35.1	1953	61.1	44.1	166.1
1973[1]	15.2	10.7	34.6	1952	67.8	48.9	188.1
1972[1,2]	18.8	14.3	38.5	1951	75.0	54.9	201.3
1971[1]	18.8	13.0	45.3	1950	83.3	61.1	221.6
1970[1]	21.5	14.4	55.9	1949	90.3	68.1	234.8
1969	22.2	15.5	55.7	1948	116.6	89.4	301.0
1968	24.5	16.6	63.6	1947	134.5	108.6	334.6
1967	28.0	19.5	69.5	1946	156.7	130.7	358.9
1966	29.1	20.2	72.4	1945	207.2	172.1	454.8
1965	31.6	21.0	83.7	1944	227.9	189.4	506.0
1964	33.3	22.3	89.9	1943	245.2	210.5	509.9
1963[3]	35.8	24.0	96.9	1942	258.7	221.8	544.0
1962[3]	35.2	23.8	95.9	1941	316.5	266.0	678.1
1961	36.9	24.9	101.3	1940	376.0	319.8	773.5
1960	37.1	26.0	97.9	1935–39	493.9	439.9	875.5
1959	37.4	25.8	102.1	1930–34[4]	636.0	575.4	1,080.7
1958	37.6	26.3	101.8	1925–29	668.6	615.0	1,163.7
1957	41.0	27.5	118.3	1920–24	689.5	649.2	1,134.5
1956	40.9	28.7	110.7	1915–19	727.9	700.3	1,253.5
1955	47.0	32.8	130.3				

[1]Excludes deaths of nonresidents of the United States.
[2]Deaths based on a 50-percent sample.
[3]Figures by color exclude data for residents of New Jersey; see Technical Appendix.
[4]For 1932–34, Mexicans are included with "All other."

Source: National Center for Health Statistics: Vital Statistics of the United States, Vol. II, Part A, 1974.

Fig. 20. Maternal mortality rates by color.

tention should be paid to nutrition. Every effort should be made to prepare the pregnant woman (and her husband) for the baby's arrival. A clear understanding of the delivery process is important and advance exposure of the primipara to the delivery room, coupled with appropriate explanation can do much to allay anxiety. In this connection, parents' classes are available in many communities, commonly sponsored by the Red Cross, hospital, or some other health agency. These classes usually consist of several sessions in which the anatomy and physiology of pregnancy and the difficulties that may occur during the course of pregnancy are discussed, as well as the delivery process and care of the newborn baby. These classes have been found to be quite useful and usually are well attended.

Pregnant women, insofar as it is possible, should be protected against communicable disease, particularly German measles, because of the hazard of the development of congenital abnormalities in the infant. Some authorities advocate exposing little girls to German measles and giving gamma globulin to women exposed to the disease during pregnancy. Special attention should be given to high-risk groups, such as women who have experienced repeated abortions or premature deliveries, or have delivered children with congenital abnormalities. High-risk patients also include those who have experienced previous difficulties during pregnancy, such as toxemia or hemorrhage, and patients who have medical complications, such as heart disease or tuberculosis.

One of the important objectives of adequate prenatal care is the prevention of prematurity. While all of the factors responsible for prematurity are not completely understood, it is believed that this may be reduced by proper medical care during pregnancy.

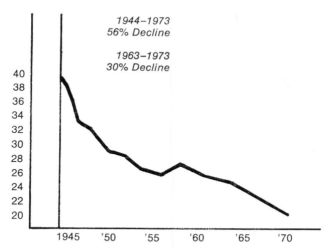

Decline in Maternal Mortality Rates

1944–1973
56% Decline

1963–1973
30% Decline

Source: The Killers and Cripplers. National Health Education Committee 1976.

Fig. 21. Crude Death Rate per 100,000 Population.

It need hardly be said that adequate provisions for receiving the pregnant woman in the hospital and for delivery of her baby in a satisfactory maternity facility are essential. The patient should receive a postpartum examination about 6 weeks after delivery. Examination of the cervix should be carried out at this time to discover erosions or chronic infections which may require treatment, as well as to detect early cancer.

While care of the pregnant woman should be carried out in the office of the physician, many health departments throughout the country have established prenatal and postnatal clinics to provide these services for those unable to afford private care. As a result of the increasing desire to use paraprofessionals, the health professions are increasingly looking to the nurse as the primary provider of care for well children, and to nurse-midwives to assume a more active role in maternity care.

FAMILY PLANNING

Interest in the area of family planning dates back many years, in fact to before this century. Community programs aimed at assisting low-income families to acquire knowledge concerning methods by which family size might be regulated have been sponsored in this country, mostly by the Planned Parenthood Association, for the past 60 years. This interest, however, has increased considerably in the past few years, and has been stimulated by a more active concern on the part of the Federal Government.

The population of the world is now growing at a rate of a little more than 2% each year. By the end of 1952 the world population was about 2.6 billion. Just 12 years later, at the end of 1964, it was 3.3 billion and by 1977 it had reached 4 billion. At the current rate, the population will reach almost 7 billion by the year 2,000. Thus, it took all of human history up to 1850 to produce a world population of 1 billion, only 75 years to reach the second billion, and just 35 years to grow to the third. These startling figures are predominately due to a marked decline in the death rate, especially during this century, primarily because of the remarkable advancements in medicine and public health that have occurred during this time. Up to the beginning of the 19th century, the average life expectancy was no more than 35 years, in any country. Today, even in the underdeveloped countries, it is often 50 years, while in this country we have achieved the Biblical three score and ten. At the current rate of population growth, it appears clear that economic and social advances will prove difficult in many countries. Even now, in countries such as India and China, it is difficult for the nation to provide sufficient food for its population. Thus the implications of the rapid surge in population are far-reaching. In the past, population growth was retarded not only by wars but particularly by the great epidemics and even endemics which decimated whole populations. Today, great advances in medicine and public health, coupled with rising standards of living, have changed this picture, so that the rapid upward march of population figures is unabated. This population growth and the attendant difficulties, nutritional, economic and social, provide the impetus for consideration of world-wide measures to control population.

Still another important social reason, however, must be considered. During the past few years, welfare rolls have continued to rise steeply, and governmental expenditures to support large indigent families have grown by leaps and bounds. Thus, it would appear evident that steps taken to provide low-income families with information and, in some cases, with the necessary materials for planning family size not only may have a beneficial effect on maternal health, but also may prevent or at least reduce dependence upon government for support.

Insofar as the United States is concerned, women who lack knowledge of birth control measures continue to give birth to additional children, even though their health has been impaired so that childbearing might prove harmful, if not hazardous. Under these common circumstances, the physician who advises his patient concerning appropriate methods to control family size is practicing good family medicine.

The birth rate has continued to decline in recent years; the 1977 rate was 15.4 per thousand population —this in spite of the fact that the number of women in the childbearing ages (15 to 44 years) has been rising rapidly as a result of high birth rates during the late 1940's and 1950's.

The largest number of abortions are reported (in States where they are legal) as having been obtained by women aged 15 to 24. Girls less than 15 or women over 40 have the highest ratios of abortions per 1,000 live births. Nearly one-half the abortions performed in 1971 were on women who had no living children. In 1969, some 13,000 legal abortions were reported. In 1977, the comparable figure was more than 1 million.

The number of teen-age pregnancies is on the increase. Most significant is the increase in pregnancies among girls under the age of 15.

Many methods of birth control are in common use today. Currently, the most popular is the contraceptive pill; the intrauterine device is popular with some, while the diaphragm, foams, jellies, condoms and the rhythm method are also used. Whichever method is selected, pelvic examination is often desirable. The wise physician will, in all cases, discuss the matter of family planning with his patient, giving due regard to her religious beliefs.

INFANT AND PRESCHOOL CHILD HEALTH

Infant Mortality

Although little progress was made in reducing infant mortality during the first half of the 1960 to 1970 period, the nation has been moving at an accelerated pace since that time in cutting infant deaths. Between 1960 and 1965, the infant mortality rate decreased only 5%

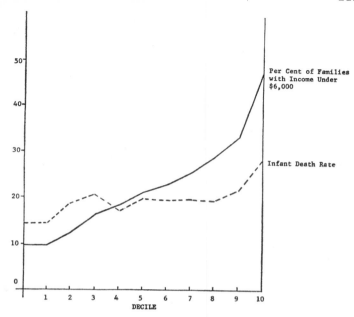

Fig. 22. Suburban Cook County by income and infant mortality. (Chicago Welfare Council Report.)

but it dropped 19% between 1965 and 1970. The rate for 1977 was 14.1 per thousand live births. Here again, however, considerable disparity exists between the rate for white (about 12) and that for black (about 22) infants. In general, the highest rates are in the lowest socioeconomic groups, both white and non-white. Approximately two-thirds of all infant deaths occur during the first month; about one-third occur on the first day of life. By far the most important factor is prematurity, followed by congenital malformations, influenza and pneumonia. While the infant mortality rate fell stead-

Cause of death	Deaths per 100,000 population	Proportion of all deaths
All causes	69.9	100.0%
Accidents	27.9	39.9
Motor vehicle	(10.5)	
All other	(17.4)	
Congenital anomalies	9.0	12.9
Malignant neoplasms	5.3	7.6
Leukemia	(2.0)	
Influenza and pneumonia	3.9	5.6
Pneumonia	(3.7)	
Cardiovascular disease	2.7	3.9
Heart disease	(1.8)	

Source: National Center for Health Statistics: Selected data from the Division of Vital Statistics

Fig. 23. Leading causes of death in children 1 to 4 years of age: United States, 1976

ily during the first half of this century, it has not fallen nearly as much since 1950; in fact, the rate has risen slightly in many large cities.

One problem which has become of serious import, particularly in recent years, concerns hospital infections with staphylococci that are resistant to antibiotics. This has occurred predominantly among newborns and may therefore produce serious consequences. The chief source of the staphylococci appears to be hospital personnel, who carry the antibiotic-resistant organisms in their noses and throats. Infected infants apparently

Country	Infant mortality rate		Average annual rate of change	Perinatal mortality ratio[2]		Average annual rate of change
	1971	1976[1]		1971	1975[3]	
	Infant deaths per 1,000 live births			Perinatal deaths per 1,000 live births		
Canada	17.6	14.3	−5.1	20.3	16.9	−5.9
United States ...	19.1	15.2	−4.5	21.9	17.9	−4.9
Sweden	11.1	8.7	−4.8	15.7	11.3	−7.9
England and Wales	17.5	14.0	−4.4	22.5	20.6	−2.9
Netherlands	12.1	10.5	−2.8	17.8	14.0	−5.8
German Demo- cratic Republic	18.0	14.1	−4.8	20.6	17.6	−3.9
German Federal Republic	23.3	17.4	−5.7	25.6	19.4	−6.7
France	17.1	12.5	−6.1	19.8	19.5	−0.5
Switzerland	14.4	10.5	−6.1	17.2	13.5	−5.9
Italy	28.5	19.1	−7.7	30.8	24.1	−5.9
Israel	20.4	22.9	2.3	22.1	20.9	−1.4
Japan	12.4	9.3	−5.6	20.3	16.0	−5.8
Australia	17.3	14.3	−4.6	—	19.2	—

[1]Data for Canada and Australia refer to 1975.
[2]Fetal deaths of 28 weeks or more gestation plus infant deaths within 7 days.
[3]Data for Canada, England and Wales, and France refer to 1974.

NOTE: Countries are grouped by continent.

SOURCES: United Nations: *Demographic Yearbook 1974 and 1976.* Pub. Nos. ST/ESA/STAT/R.3 and ST/ESA/STAT/SER.R/4. New York. United Nations, 1975 and 1977; World Health Organization: *World Health Statistics, 1977,* Vol. 1. Geneva. World Health Organization, 1977; World Health Organization: Selected data.

Fig. 24. Infant mortality rates and perinatal mortality ratios: Selected countries, selected years 1971–76 (Data are based on national vital registration systems)

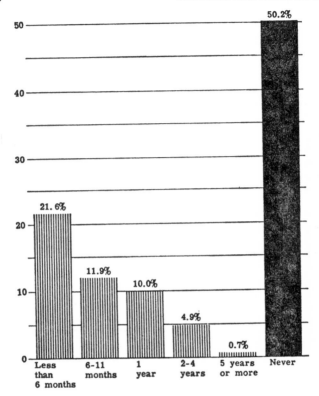

Fig. 25. Half of the children under 15 in the United States have never been to a dentist. (New York Academy of Medicine Health Conference, December, 1965.)

then spread the disease to others in the newborn nursery and to their mothers. The first sign of the disease usually occurs in the infants shortly after they are discharged from the hospital. The mothers may soon develop breast abscesses, and the disease may spread to other members of the family and persist in the family for a considerable time.

Control of this problem usually requires careful surveillance by a hospital infection committee, with careful development of hospital policies and control of carriers found in the hospital. The local health department can play an important role because of their familiarity with epidemiologic methods and environmental health programs.

Preschool Child Mortality

There has been a considerable decline in mortality rates in the 1 to 4 year age group over the past half century, primarily due to a decrease in deaths from communicable diseases. At present the commonest cause of death in this age group is accidents. While mortality is relatively low in this group, morbidity, however, is quite high. In addition, this is a time of growth and development, both physical and emotional. Emphasis, therefore, is placed upon health maintenance and promotion, perhaps more than on prevention of death.

Lead Poisoning in Children

This results mostly from ingestion of chips of lead-containing paint from walls and woodwork in old dilapidated houses. Its etiology, pathogenesis, pathophysiology, and epidemiology are known. Practical methods are available for screening, diagnosis, prevention and treatment. Yet each year, lead poisoning continues to cause the deaths of many children and mental retardation or other neurological handicaps in many other children. Although slum areas in large, old cities have by far the greatest incidence, it has also been reported in children from economically and socially advantaged homes. However, high risk areas for lead poisoning are almost synonymous with the slums where old, dilapidated houses prevail. In these areas, accessibility to flaking paint and broken plaster, together with lack of adequate parental supervision, provides an optimum environment for lead poisoning. Here, dwellings often have several coats of paint on walls, woodwork and ceilings, and the base coats generally contain significant amounts of lead.

Children between the ages of 1 and 6 years are the main victims; those between 1 and 3 years of age comprise approximately 85% of the cases. Across the United States, 25,800 confirmed cases were reported in fiscal 1978. In New York City alone, 3,295 confirmed cases of lead poisoning in children were reported in that year. In Baltimore, during the period 1956 to 1964, there were 1,337 known cases. In Cleveland, the mortality rate reported for lead poisoning from 1952 to 1958 was 30%. For many of those who survive, the outlook is grim. In Chicago, a study of 425 children who were followed for 6 months to 10 years after treatment for lead poisoning revealed that 39% had some kind of neurologic sequelae.

Clearly, the most important single preventive is provided by clearing cities of old dilapidated houses. Educational programs directed to the public and to physicians are also important. Public health nurses, in their home visits, can play a key role with low income families in slum areas. Facilities for early recognition, diagnosis, and early treatment are obviously indicated, particularly in large cities. In some instances, screening programs using blood lead determinations have been set up for children ages 1 to 6 years from high risk areas.

Infant and Preschool Child Health Services

Prematurity. A premature birth is usually defined as a live-born infant weighing 2500 grams or less at birth. Approximately 8.8% of all births in the United States are premature. While deaths from this cause have fallen in the past half century, this reduction has not been nearly as great as the reduction of deaths from other causes. Thus, prematurity is assuming an increasing relative importance as a cause of infant and neonatal deaths. One-third of all infant deaths are, in fact, a result of prematurity. While the exact cause of prematurity is unknown in many cases, a considerable number are associated with conditions such as toxemia of pregnancy, placenta praevia, hypertension and multiple pregnancies. Early recognition of multiple pregnancy makes possible more intensive prenatal care and, therefore, can contribute to the prevention of prematurity. Similarly, early effective prenatal care may reduce toxemia, while birth-control measures may be indicated in the presence of chronic hypertension in a woman. Early case finding and thorough treatment of syphilis will prevent prematurity from this cause. Certainly, early adequate prenatal care is the essential ingredient in all of these preventive measures.

In dealing with the premature infant, it must be recognized that the premature child has a higher risk of death and of developing handicapping conditions than does the full-term baby. Consequently, special care is needed in caring for the premature infant. Thus, hospitals must be adequately equipped and staffed to provide the "round-the-clock" care that the infant may require. In fact, if a hospital does not possess these resources, it may be better to transport the infant, in an incubator, to a hospital where the necessary facilities

6

and staff are available. In any event, the premature baby should not be cared for at home, at least for the first month or so. Good nursing care is essential, particularly in the first few days of life, and it is difficult, if not impossible, to provide all of these services in a private home.

One of the major hazards affecting both premature and full-term babies is possible infection. Stringent steps must be taken to avoid the introduction and spread of infection in the newborn nursery.

Well-Baby Care. One of the most important pediatric services is that revolving around the routine care of the well infant and young child. In well-baby care, much good preventive medicine can be practiced during the child's important formative years. An excellent opportunity is provided for the child to be maintained under constant surveillance, to receive regular physical examinations aimed at revealing any untoward defects and immunization against such diseases as diphtheria, pertussis, tetanus, smallpox, poliomyelitis, measles and rubella. Moreover, such care affords a fine opportunity for the parents to discuss their child with a physician, who can play an important role during this period in allaying many fears associated with parenthood. The infant's nutritional status can be observed and appropriate dietary changes may be recommended. Early evidence of illness can be detected, and diagnostic tests and treatment initiated at an early date. Tuberculin testing can be performed, as well as screening tests for visual or hearing defects.

In many communities, health departments have established public well-baby clinics to provide well-baby services to families who find it difficult to pay for these services privately. These clinics are almost always popular and, in most cases, public agencies find it difficult to keep up with the demand for them. One of their disadvantages is related to the fact that during an acute illness the child would be under the care of a physician different from the one who cared for him when he was well.

THE SCHOOL CHILD

Death rates in the age group 5 to 14 years are also rather low; by far the commonest cause of death is, again, accidents. Just as in the preschool group, however, this is an important period of growth and development. Therefore, the emphasis in terms of preventive medicine is on promotion of health rather than prevention of mortality.

School Health Services

While it is true that mortality in age group 5 to 14 is low, these are important years in the child's growth and development, both physical and emotional, and it is, therefore, in these areas that much emphasis is placed during this period. It is also a time during which the child has a particular desire to learn and it is, therefore, a time when effort may be directed at teaching him some of the fundamental principles involved in personal hygiene and in the protection of health.

Most communities in this country have fairly well-organized publicly financed school health programs, usually administered by either the health department or the board of education, or jointly. The most important single objective of his program is aimed at ensuring that no child is prevented by some physical or emotional health defect from taking advantage of the educational opportunities offered him. It is clear, for example, that a child with poor vision may have difficulty in reading what the teacher has placed on the blackboard; similarly, the child with a hearing defect may fail to achieve suitable grades in school. For these reasons, screening for vision and hearing defects is commonly carried out as part of the school health program. Those failing the screening test are usually referred for private medical care (or to public facilities when the family is indigent).

At one time, many school systems required annual physical examinations of all school children. This procedure, however, has not been found to be particularly fruitful, and the basis for many programs today revolves around the teacher-nurse conference. This is a meeting between the teacher and the school nurse during which the more obvious health defects observed by the teacher are discussed. Referral for appropriate diagnosis and, if necessary, treatment is then made.

Because many children of school age exhibit behavior disorders and other emotional problems, mental health consultation is usually provided as part of the school health program. A considerable number of children also have speech defects, so that speech therapy is also a necessary part of the program.

Gonorrhea has been rising markedly in children and adolescents. Most States now permit physicians to examine and treat minors for venereal diseases on their own consent (without requiring parental permission).

The special health problems of the adolescent such as drug abuse, pregnancies, venereal diseases and psycho-social problems are receiving increasing attention from health programs at the national, state, and local levels. There is growing recognition, too, that some health problems in later life have their beginnings in these early years. For example, some authorities now believe that adult arteriosclerosis will be understood and controlled only through an understanding of its pathogenesis in adolescence.

Health programs in school, whether concerned with screening for defects, the initiation of tuberculin testing programs, communicable disease control, dental services or any other activity, should be accompanied by health education aimed at providing the children with a simple understanding of the health subject involved. For example, screening for hearing defects might well be preceded by some explanation of the anatomy and physiology of the ear.

Environmental health programs in a school system also form a part of the usual school health program. Adequate toilet facilities, water supply, heating, lighting and ventilation, together with the elimination of accident hazards wherever possible, are all important.

The physician in practice can often play an important role in the school health program. He will receive referrals of patients and will be requested to report back to the school his findings and recommendations. He will also be called upon frequently to indicate whether a child has a communicable disease and whether a child should or should not be in school. In all cases, a physician should take time out to acquaint himself with the applicable laws and regulations in the area in which he practices; many difficulties could be avoided if this were done. In some cases, the physician may be called upon to carry out physical examinations of selected children in the school itself.

SERVICES FOR HANDICAPPED CHILDREN

Community organized and administered programs dealing with handicapped children are quite extensive in many parts of the United States. While many voluntary health agencies, civic organizations and service clubs have, for many years, provided financial support for such programs, tax-supported services developed substantially after passage of the Social Security Act of 1935, which authorized the use of federal funds for services to crippled children. The total grant to States in 1935 was 1.2 million dollars. By 1972, this figure had increased to more than 62 million dollars. The States are required to match this federal money in varying degrees. The objective of this program, then, as now, was to locate handicapped children and to provide medical, surgical, and rehabilitative services and facilities for them. Federal financial support for this program is administered by the Department of Health and Human Services.

While accurate data on the number of children suffering from various handicapping conditions are difficult to secure, the following rough estimates of prevalence of certain handicaps among children below 21 years of age may serve to indicate how frequent these conditions are.

Handicap	*Prevalence per 100 Children*
Emotional Problems	10
Mental Retardation	3
Orthopedic Problems	2
Cardiac Defects	1
Speech Defects	2
Hearing Defects	1
Cerebral Palsy	0.5
Epilepsy	0.5

Obviously, children with handicapping conditions require health supervision as do normal children; they require immunizations, counselling, etc. In fact, they may require more intensive health supervision than will the normal child because their handicap may make them more susceptible to disease. The first important need in a community program for handicapped children is for case finding. Case detection should be started as early as possible, for example, at birth or during infancy. Subsequently, defects may be located during routine well-baby care or as part of the school health program. In all cases, adequate diagnostic facilities should be provided to aid the private physician who may not be able to establish clearly an accurate diagnosis alone on some conditions, such as mental retardation, congenital heart disease, or emotional disorder. Adequate treatment and rehabilitation staff and facilities should also be provided. For example, while the physician obviously plays an important part in the diagnosis and treatment of crippled children, many other disciplines need to be involved. Children with hearing and speech disorders require the skill not only of an otolaryngologist, but also of a speech therapist, audiologist and sometimes a psychologist or psychiatrist. In many communities, particularly in some of our major urban centers, centrally located diagnostic and treatment facilities may exist, particularly in university settings or in major hospitals. At these centers, a range of professional skills and diagnostic and treatment facilities are available. These can be of tremendous assistance to the physician.

Many handicapping conditions, of course, can be prevented. For example, deafness is often preventable. Measures taken to prevent prematurity or brain injury, prompt treatment of syphilis in pregnant women, and early and thorough treatment of otitis media are all examples of preventive methods. So, too, are safety precautions involving fireworks and sliding glass doors as well as prophylactic treatment of the eyes of newborn babies in blindness prevention. Thorough treatment of streptococcal sore throat may prevent rheumatic fever and rheumatic heart disease.

REFERENCES

Altenderfer, M. D., and Crowther, B.: Relationships between infant mortality and socio-economic factors in urban areas, Pub. Health Rep. 64:331, 1949.

American Public Health Association: Health Supervision of Young Children, New York, 1955.

Brown, B. S.: Regarding the emergency room (correspondence), New Eng. J. Med. 258:507, 1958.

Eliot, M. M.: Deaths around birth—The National score, J.A.M.A. 167:945, 1958.

Gray, S. E.: *Community Health Today,* New York, The Macmillan Co., 1978.

Haggerty, R. J., and Roghmann, K. J.: Pless I-V *Child Health and the Community,* New York, John C. Wiley Co., 1975.

Harper, P. A.: *Preventive Pediatrics, Child Health and Development,* New York, Appleton-Century-Crofts, Inc., 1962.

Lead Poisoning in Children, Public Health Service Publication 2108, U.S. Department of HEW, 1970.

Promoting the Health of Mothers and Children, U.S. Department of HEW, 1972.

The Population Council 1952-1964, A Report, New York, July, 1965.

U.S. Department of Health, Education & Welfare, Public Health Service, Vital and Health Statistics, *The Change in Mortality Trends in the United States,* Series 3, No. 1, March, 1964.

Chapter 9

Food and Nutrition

While it is true that, at least in this country, it is quite rare to find severe acute nutritional deficiency diseases such as scurvy, beriberi or pellagra, dietary studies have clearly shown that a substantial proportion of our population is deficient to some degree in one or more nutrients. Furthermore, if we accept the relationship between obesity, disease and longevity, there is little question that this aspect of nutrition is one which requires considerable attention. In addition, technologic advances have brought about great changes in the nutritional values of commonly consumed food products through advances in processing, transportation, storage, enrichment and fortification. Examples include the addition of vitamin D to milk, B vitamins and iron to cereals, flour and bread, and vitamin A to margarine.

The eating habits of people are greatly influenced by social and cultural traditions, by emotional factors, and by environment. In general, knowledge of nutritional value plays a small role in determining what people will consume. Great variations in eating habits are found not only among different ethnic groups, but in different regions of the country and among different social classes. In many cases, inexpensive foods are rejected without any reference to their nutritional value which often is as high as in the most expensive items. Religious customs also play an important role in determining whether or not certain foods are consumed.

It must also be understood that nutrition includes not only the ingestion of desirable nutrients through proper quantities of foods, but also their digestion and absorption by the body, transport to the tissues and utilization by the cells. Impairment of nutrition can result from interference with any stage of this process.

Normal Nutritional Requirements

Caloric Intake. The number of calories a person requires depends essentially upon his basal metabolism plus his degree of physical activity, although age, sex, body size and climatic conditions are also factors. Thus, the Committee on Foods and Nutrition of the National Research Council recommends a 2900 calorie intake for an average-sized, physically active 25-year-old man, and 2100 calories for an active woman of the same age but of lesser weight. The requirements of an adolescent boy are usually greater than those for a grown man, whereas elderly persons do not usually require as many calories as do younger individuals.

Protein. Protein requirement is particularly important during the growth periods of life, namely, for infants, children and adolescents, when rapid development of tissues takes place. Protein is needed for growth and regeneration of tissues and is therefore particularly important during pregnancy and lactation. Since it is the most expensive of all food elements, a reduced intake of protein is often found with economic stress. Protein deficiency is particularly common, therefore, in underdeveloped areas of the world.

Carbohydrates and Fats. Carbohydrates, the cheapest form of food, constitute the most efficient source of energy for the body and usually comprise more than half of the usual diet. Fats are a highly concentrated source of energy and often contain appreciable quantities of fat-soluble vitamins. Fat consumption in the United States tends to be higher than that of many other countries. It is thought that persons with high blood cholesterol may be able to reduce this to some extent by maintaining a low-fat diet.

Minerals. Many minerals are essential to the human body. Calcium, for example, is an essential ingredient of bones and teeth and is particularly important during pregnancy and lactation. Iron is an essential ingredient of the blood and is urgently needed by women because of blood loss during menstruation; it is also important during pregnancy.

Vitamins. While a great deal of knowledge concerning vitamins and the human body's requirements has accumulated, much still remains to be acquired. In general, vitamins may be water soluble, such as the B vitamins and vitamin C, or fat-soluble, as is the case with vitamins A and D. In the United States, varying degrees of vitamin deficiency occur with considerable frequency, although frank deficiency such as beriberi and scurvy is rarely seen. It is also possible to have too high a vitamin intake; this appears to be particularly the case with vitamins A and D.

Malnutrition

Malnutrition may include any type of nutritional disorder in an individual and embraces over-indulgence as well as deficiency. It may be caused by one or more factors.

Factors Increasing Body Requirements. Caloric requirements vary with the degree of physical activity; protein needs are particularly great in infants and children; calcium and iron are urgently needed by pregnant women, while vitamin D is essential for bone development in infants and children. Anything that increases body metabolism will raise the nutrient requirements. Thus, fever increases the demand for nutrients. Furthermore, since fever is often associated with anorexia, vomiting or diarrhea, weight loss may be severe.

Factors Interfering with Ingestion of Food. Among the most important factors in this category are those dealing with inability to buy adequate nutrients, as well as the social and cultural patterns which may have a profound effect upon food intake. Perhaps the most serious nutritional deficiency in the world today is kwashiorkor. This disease occurs in infants and small children and results from a diet high in carbohydrates and low in protein following weaning. It occurs particularly in sections of the world where economic conditions render the purchase of protein difficult, or even impossible. The disease produces changes in the color of the hair, skin lesions, diarrhea, edema and enlarged liver.

Other factors which may reduce food intake include loss of appetite, such as occurs in many diseases and in alcoholism, or when a person is in pain; neurologic and psychiatric disorders and other handicapping conditions which may interfere with the process of self-feeding; loss of teeth, gastrointestinal disorders and special therapeutic diets (such as those necessitated by food allergies) which purposefully restrict the intake of certain foods.

Factors Interfering with Digestion or Absorption of Food. Atrophy of the intestinal tract resulting from inadequate intake of vitamins of the B complex will produce interference with absorption of food. In diarrhea, the passage of food is hastened through the intestinal tract giving insufficient time for adequate absorption. Treatment of peptic ulcer with alkalis may interfere with the digestive and absorptive processes. A high pH of the gastric juices may destroy certain vitamins.

Factors Interfering with Utilization of Nutrients by the Tissues. In thyroid disease, there may be failure on the part of the thyroid gland to pick up iodine; in disease of the kidney or liver, vitamin A will not be properly utilized, while in adrenal disease, vitamin C may not be picked up. In cirrhosis of the liver there may be interference with the conversion of carotene to vitamin A.

Factors Increasing Excretion. Excessive protein loss may result from hemorrhage, burns or injuries; an increased fluid output may occur in fevers, polyuria and lactation, while various drugs may increase the excretion of certain nutrients. Increased excretion may also occur in diabetes.

Dietary Management During Pregnancy

Over most of recorded history, special attention has been given to the diets of pregnant women. Some kinds of food have been restricted, while others have been regarded as necessary to prevent hazards to the mother or infant.

An average weight gain during pregnancy, of 24 pounds, is commensurate with a better than average course and outcome of pregnancy. There is no scientific justification for limitation of weight gain to lesser amounts. Severe caloric restriction is potentially hazardous to the developing fetus and to the mother and almost inevitably restricts other nutrients essential for growth processes. Weight reduction regimes, if needed, should be instituted only after pregnancy is terminated.

The young adolescent poses special problems during pregnancy. Her own growth requires an adequate diet with particular reference to calories, protein and calcium, and she tolerates caloric deprivation poorly. Therefore, when the nutritional demands of pregnancy are superimposed on those of adolescence, there should be no stringent caloric restriction.

Special attention should be paid to the dietary intake and food habits of women who enter pregnancy in a poor nutritional state. Young adolescents, women who have been on slimming regimens, and those of low socioeconomic status are particularly vulnerable to the metabolic demands of pregnancy.

Vitamin and mineral supplements should not be routinely instituted as a means for correcting poor food habits. In considering the wisdom of recommending them, the relative cost, as compared to enhancing the nutrient intake with foods, should be taken into account, especially in caring for pregnant women with inadequate incomes.

In view of the rather frequent incidence of nutritional anemia and the increased iron requirements of pregnancy, iron supplementation is needed during the second and third trimesters.

Nutrition of Infancy

Formula or milk ordinarily accounts for a major proportion of the total calories and essential nutrients during the first 2 years of life. During the first few months, the entire caloric intake may well be from formula;

however, nowadays, many parents add solid foods to the diet during the first month or two of life so that by 6 months of age most infants receive approximately one-third of their calories from foods other than milk or formula.

In order to assure a reasonable distribution of calories from protein, carbohydrates and fat, it is generally desirable to continue the feeding of formula until the carbohydrate supplied by other food is sufficient to compensate for carbohydrate previously contributed by the formula.

Human milk and commercially prepared infant formula usually provide adequate intakes of ascorbic acid. Whole cow's milk and evaporated milk does not supply adequate amounts of ascorbic acid; therefore, infants fed these milks should receive supplementary ascorbic acid in the form of a drop preparation, or in fresh, frozen, or canned fruit juices.

The Recommended Dietary Allowance of vitamin D during infancy is that amount present in a 13-fluid ounce can of evaporated milk or in a quart of vitamin D fortified whole milk.

Human milk and cow's milk are both poor sources of iron; thus a source of iron should be added to the infant's diet in early infancy. Similarly, both human's milk and cow's milk are poor sources of fluoride. Whether or not a fluoride supplement should be given to an infant will depend upon how much water the infant consumes and whether or not that water supply contains fluoride.

During the second and third years of life, the child grows much less rapidly than during the first year. It is nevertheless important to continue providing those foods which help to meet the child's needs for growth and activity.

Obesity

While it is generally true that the average person in this country does not gauge his food intake according to nutritional requirements, the subject of obesity has become a popular topic of conversation and many individuals, particularly women, spend considerable time trying out various methods designed to reduce weight.

While there may be difficulty in recognizing nutritional deficiencies in an individual, obesity generally is only too obvious and may become a source of embarrassment.

It should be understood that a person cannot be obese without being overweight, but he may be overweight without being obese. On the other hand, it is true, of course, that a person who is considerably overweight is likely to be obese, at least to some degree. The studies carried out by life insurance companies, however, deal specifically with the subject of weight, not necessarily obesity. They have revealed a close relationship between excess weight and reduced life span. A study of 5,000,000 insured persons showed a one-third greater mortality among males between the ages of 15 and 69 years who were 20% or more overweight than among males of the same age range who were of normal or subnormal weight. According to these studies, in the United States, approximately 20% of persons over 20 years of age are 10% overweight. The excess mortality referred to above appears to be primarily due to diabetes, digestive system diseases, cardiovascular disease and cancer.

In the treatment of obesity, it is important to take off the excess fat at such a rate and in such a manner that the body is not harmed and the individual can continue to function at a reasonable level. A daily caloric deficit of 500 calories will permit a loss of approximately 1 pound per week. The value of a moderate increase in exercise as a means of increasing energy output and reducing weight should also be kept in mind for some individuals.

The Detection and Handling of Malnutrition

It is by no means a simple matter to detect evidence of malnutrition. The frank deficiency diseases, underweight or overweight, are usually obvious. Outright beriberi, scurvy or pellagra usually can be diagnosed readily. But, in the United States, the presence of a degree of deficiency in one or more nutrients that is not sufficiently severe to cause easily recognizable symptoms is often difficult to detect. It will usually require investigation into the food intake habits of the individual followed by an analysis of the nutritional value of these foods as related to the individual's needs. Thus, a knowledge of the nutritional composition of foods is essential. These data are then correlated with clinical and laboratory findings before a decision can be reached as to whether or not dietary changes are advisable.

A change in diet must take into account the individual's ability to purchase the foods recommended, his food likes and habits, and religious, ethnic, social and cultural factors that may influence his willingness to follow a recommended diet. The role of disease in producing malnutrition must be recognized, and appropriate steps are necessary to ensure an adequate supply of needed nutrients, by either regular food intake or the use of dietary supplements.

Prevention of Malnutrition

Malnutrition in the United States is usually the result of poor judgment in budgetary expenditures for

Food and Nutrition

food, failure to understand the importance of proper nutrition in growth and development, lack of knowledge concerning basic nutritional requirements and failure to recognize nutritional deficiencies when they occur. The correction of this situation requires a close working relationship between the private physician and various community health agencies with the objectives of:

1. Understanding of basic food needs.
2. Correction of improper food habits in children, together with appropriate instruction of parents concerning food requirements for their infants and children
3. Provision for the special requirements of the prenatal and maternal period
4. Special diet instruction for certain categories of patients such as diabetics or those with food allergies
5. Assistance with food budgeting, menu planning and food preparation
6. Proper use of community resources such as the school lunch program or food stamp plan.

REFERENCES

Browe, J. H.: Provision of Suitable and Sufficient Nutrition, in *Preventive Medicine,* Hilleboe and Larimore, 2nd Ed., Philadelphia, W. B. Saunders Co., 1965.

Cassel, J.: Social & Cultural Implications of Food and Food Habits, Amer. J. Publ. Health 47:732, 1957.

Food and Nutrition Board, Recommended Dietary Allowances; National Academy of Sciences—National Research Council, Publication No. 1146, Washington, D.C. 1964.

Goodhart, R. S. and Shils, M. E.: *Modern Nutrition in Health and Disease,* 6th Ed., Philadelphia, Lea & Febiger, 1980.

Maternal Nutrition and the Course of Pregnancy, U.S. Department of HEW, 1970.
Nutrition and Feeding of Infants and Children Under Three in Group Day Care, U.S. Department of HEW, 1971.
Scrimshaw, N. S.: Ecological Factors in Nutrition Disease, Amer. J. Clin. Nutrition, *14*:112, 1964.

Chapter 10

Dental Health

Extent of the Problem

Practically no individual in the course of a lifetime escapes dental disease. The civilian population of the United States currently spends approximately 10% of its total medical care expenditures on dental health. The most common cause of rejection for Selective Service of the first two million men called in 1941 was dental defects. Almost 10% of those examined were rejected because of such defects. It has been estimated that some 75% of children entering school have evidence of dental caries. The U.S. National Health Survey carried out in 1957 and 1958 revealed some 13% of the population to be edentulous; for persons aged 35 and over, the rate was 29%.

In spite of these indications of the extensive prevalence of dental disease, and even though the United States ranks high in dentist-population ratio, our present complement of dentists does not seem able to cope adequately with this enormous problem. As a matter of fact, the ratio of dentists to patients has declined over the past 50 years. In 1930, in the United States there was one dentist for every 1700 persons. In 1980, this ratio was 1 for 2400. On the other hand, in 1930, some 20 to 25% of the population received some dental care. By 1969, approximately 45% of the population received regular dental care as represented by an average of 3.8 visits per person per year. Clearly, auxiliaries have played an important role.

It has been estimated that children in the United States receive care for about a fifth of their dental needs. While the increasing use of dental hygienists and assistants has unquestionably helped the dental manpower problem, it has by no means solved it. Nor, of course, has it had any appreciable influence on the ability of many individuals to be able to afford dental care. Unfortunately, too, while great strides have been made in the availability of health insurance plans for medical and hospital care, this has not been true of dental care; only a few dental insurance programs are available, and some of these leave much to be desired.

Over 50% of all children under age 15 have never been to a dentist. Almost 70% of the children in poor families have never been to a dentist.

Cleft palate, with or without cleft lip, occurs about once in every 700 births.

Oral cancer is discovered in 14,000 new patients each year and accounts for over 7,000 deaths yearly. Of those who have had treatment, approximately 22% are in need of maxillofacial prosthesis.

There are many reasons why people do not seek regular dental care. These include financial barriers, lack of understanding of the value of good dental health, fear of pain, and the inconvenience of going to the dentist. The most important of these is cost. Many people cannot afford dental care because they have no financial method available to budget the cost.

Large numbers of our people, not having sought reg-

Persons with no, one, or both arches edentulous, according to sex and age: United States, 1971–74

(Data are based on physical examinations of a sample of the civilian non-institutionalized population)

| | Population in thousands | Per cent with | | |
		No arch edentulous	One arch edentulous	Both arches edentulous
Both sexes				
6–74 years	177,028	82.6	6.7	10.7
6–11 years	23,356	99.9	0.0	0.0
12–17 years ...	24,654	99.7	0.2	0.1
18–44 years ...	73,882	90.3	5.6	4.1
45–64 years ...	42,362	62.7	13.5	23.8
65–74 years ...	12,774	39.1	15.4	45.5
Male[1]				
6–74 years	84,644	84.7	5.7	9.5
6–11 years	11,797	99.9	0.1	0.0
12–17 years ...	12,401	100.0	—	—
18–44 years ...	34,917	92.1	4.5	3.4
45–64 years ...	20,073	65.3	12.2	22.5
65–74 years ...	5,456	40.9	15.5	43.6
Female[1]				
6–74 years	90,638	80.6	7.6	11.8
6–11 years	11,368	100.0	—	—
12–17 years ...	12,045	99.4	0.3	0.3
18–44 years ...	37,945	88.7	6.6	4.7
45–64 years ...	22,025	60.4	14.7	24.9
65–74 years ...	7,255	37.7	15.3	47.9

[1]Population of males and females include only white and black persons. Persons other than white or black are included in the both sexes category.

SOURCE: Division of Health Examination Statistics, National Center for Health Statistics: Data from the Health Nutrition Examination Survey.

ular dental care for financial reasons, inaccessibility of dentists, or other factors, are faced by emergencies requiring an unexpected, large outlay of cash to repair the accumulated damage done to their teeth and supporting structures.

The seeking of dentists' services is related to the educational and income level of the family, the availability of dental service, and the effectiveness and organization of dental programs. The relationship of family income to dental care is indicated by the finding that 66% of children in families with incomes under $4,000 have never been to a dentist, compared to 40% of children from families with incomes of $4,000 or more.

Utilization of dentists' services can be increased by removing or reducing financial barriers as demonstrated by the experience of dental prepayment programs. Utilization was increased to 70% in a program for children which included a periodic recall system. An effective program of dental health education can also increase utilization.

Dimensions of Dental Health Problem

Fewer than half the people in this country have dental examinations or treatment in a given year and far fewer than that receive dental care on a regular basis.

By age 2, 50% of America's children have decayed teeth. On entering school, the average child has three decayed teeth and by age 15, the average child has 11 teeth decayed, missing, or filled.

About half of the school-age children in America suffer from gingivitis, which can lead to progressive periodontal disease, a major cause of tooth loss in adults.

The dental profession in the United States has forcefully insisted that dental health, as an integral part of total health, be given high priority in all health programs. In the process, the value of dental health to general health should also be reassessed because too frequently dental care has been considered a fringe benefit rather than an integral part of health care.

A few cities have programs of dental inspection in schools with referrals to dentists or checkups by a dental hygienist, but these also are neither numerous nor far-reaching. The board of education, the board of health, the welfare department, or a local hospital may operate the program. The variation in mechanisms of payment, number of pupils covered, services provided, and methods of administration is extraordinary.

Inasmuch as communities have approached the dental health problem piecemeal and most of them have paid no attention to it at all, the programs may cover educational materials, limited dental care, or preventive services, but frequently cover none of these. A comprehensive program for all those eligible in any age group under public auspices does not exist. Although the priorities vary considerably, depending on the purpose of the plan, the dominant emphasis in all of them is on the importance of preventive dentistry, and the first priority of treatment is for younger age groups.

The most economic and efficient way of improving the nation's dental health is to prevent dental disease. Dental caries, periodontal disease, and oral cancer can largely be prevented, but we have failed to apply fully the preventive measures at hand. Fluoridation, for example, prevents as much as 65% of tooth decay; it is safe, economical, and simple to implement. It is an ideal health measure, yet after more than 50 years of study and nearly three decades of practical experience, this country has succeeded in fluoridating the drinking water of only half of its population. Only one of four public water supplies has been fluoridated. Fluoridation is also a proven economy. It cuts the cost of treating tooth decay among schoolchildren in half and its preventive benefits last a lifetime.

Periodontal disease can be prevented and successfully controlled when detected early and treated promptly. Although preventive periodontal measures are more complicated and less well demonstrated than fluoridation, there is sufficient knowledge to begin preventive public health periodontal programs.

Most, if not all, new victims of oral cancer could be successfully treated if such conditions were detected early and treated immediately. A sustained oral cancer detection program by all dentists is essential.

Variations in the alignment of teeth range from minimal deviations to handicapping malocclusions. If they are detected early and treated properly during the growth and development years, many serious malocclusions can be minimized or prevented by orthodontic measures that control adverse factors to dentofacial growth and guide the developing dentition.

Dental disease in the United States is almost universal. Despite an estimated $8.6 billion expenditure in fiscal year 1976, a substantial portion of the nation's dental care needs are unmet. The Department of Health, Education, and Welfare's Health and Nutrition Examination Survey conducted between 1971 and 1974 showed that 65% of the population had untreated dental problems. Blacks and low income groups experienced higher rates of untreated oral problems. Forty-five per cent of the population between the ages of 65 and 75 years were edentulous.

A survey conducted by the Department of Health, Education, and Welfare's Center for Health Statistics in 1977 disclosed that only some 50% of the American people had visited a dentist in the previous 12 months and that 50 million had never visited a dentist. American industry loses over 100 million man hours of production time annually because of problems related to dental health.

According to a national dental report there are about 1 billion unfilled dental cavities in the United States today. Half of the school-age population has some form of malocclusion and gingival disease. Each year more than 6,000 babies are born with cleft lip or palate, and oral cancer strikes some 14,000 of our people, causing 1 in every 40 deaths from cancer.

Dentists who examine new recruits entering the armed services of the United States see a pageant of dental neglect. Those dentists report that every 100 recruits minimally require 500 fillings, 80 extractions, 25 dental bridges, and 20 dentures.

Although statistics only outline the national problem, they lead to the conclusion that known preventive measures are not being fully applied. Millions of Americans receive only emergency care or no care at all, and the current dental force now provides adequate dental care to less than half the total population.

Dental diseases affect almost everyone. Dental diseases are not self-healing and cannot be cured by drugs or advice alone. Most dental diseases are irreversible and become more severe without treatment. Even with treatment, dental problems often recur and one defect compounds another. Dental problems have become so common and widespread that people apparently accept them and tooth loss as inevitable.

Twenty-five million people in the United States are completely without natural teeth; three of ten people past age 35; four of ten people past age 45; five of ten people past age 55. Eighty-six per cent of all tooth loss results from caries and periodontal disease.

There is a tendency to accept dental disease complacently because of the undramatic nature of most dental problems. The casual acceptance of dental disease probably contributes to the postponement of visiting the dentist, along with other factors such as fear of treatment and the cost of care. These barriers prevent many people from seeking the professional services they need and from enjoying the benefits of good oral health.

The mouth serves not only the essential functions of speech and appearance, but is also the center of taste, mastication, and certain digestive functions. The mouth registers personality and expression of feelings and is the principal means of communicating with the world. It is a cardinal esthetic feature of every individual and a unique sensual and psychological entity as well.

Dental Caries

Dental caries, one of the most prevalent diseases of mankind, occur when the following factors are present:

1. Susceptibility—The enamel of the teeth is decalcified by acids formed from the degradation of fermentable carbohydrates in the mouth. On the other hand, it is well known that there are some people who are essentially immune to caries. It is believed that this is probably due to resistance of the enamel of their teeth to the caries process.
2. Presence of fermentable carbohydrates—The most common types of fermentable carbohydrates are sugars and refined starch.
3. Presence of oral microorganisms capable of carbohydrate degradation—Studies of animals raised in a sterile environment have revealed that it is not pos-

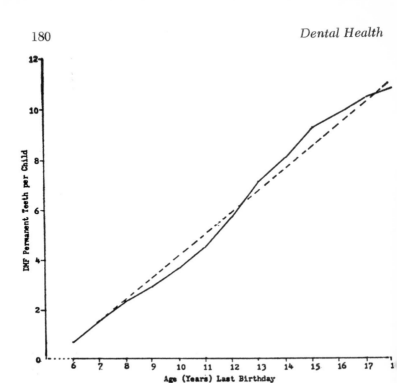

Fig. 26. Decayed, missing and filled permanent teeth per child, by age. (Sartwell: *Preventive Medicine and Public Health,* Maxcy and Rosenau (Eds.) 10th Ed., New York, Appleton-Century-Crofts.)

sible to produce caries in these animals despite their being fed a high carbohydrate diet.

Caries formation begins early in life. It has been estimated that by age 1 year, as many as 5% of children have one or more carious teeth. In a study of preschool children in New York State, it was found that over 75% of 5-year-olds had some caries experience. It can be estimated that in general, a child will then average one new carious tooth each year. By about 17 years of age, almost all children will have had one or more carious permanent teeth. The Selective Service examinations carried out in 1941 showed that almost 10% of the men examined did not have 12 sound teeth in good condition out of a possible complement of 32. Almost all of this was due to dental caries. The disease tends to be more common in females than in males, and there is strong evidence of an inherited susceptibility.

Prevention

There are three major techniques to be used in the prevention of dental caries:

1. The restriction of fermentable carbohydrates in the diet—Certainly anything which reduces the amount of sweet foods ingested should have an effect on reducing dental caries. It is also questionable, however, whether any community-wide campaign urging widespread reduction in the intake of sweet foods can be really successful at the present time.
2. The observation of good mouth hygiene—This can be accomplished primarily by brushing the teeth immediately after eating or drinking any food. While there is little question that this practice, which has the effect of removing fermentable foodstuff from the teeth before degradation can take place, is of great value in reducing dental caries, it is of limited value for general use because it appears to be impractical to a large extent.
3. Use of fluoride solutions—The use of topical fluoride directly applied to the teeth in the dentist's office appears to be of considerable value in reducing dental caries. On the other hand, the most widely

used of the prophylactic fluoridation techniques involves fluoridation of public water supplies. Repeated studies have shown that one part fluoride to a million parts water is effective in reducing dental caries by as much as 60%. One of the best studies of this kind is the Newburgh-Kingston study, carried out in the state of New York, beginning in 1945, and mentioned in the chapter "Principles of Epidemiology." Many communities in the United States have since added fluoride to their water supply. There is no question that this is the single, best, most economical and most practical method known to prevent dental caries.

Because of the widespread prevalence of dental caries, regular visits to the dentist, preferably twice a year, are desirable so that the caries can be removed and the infected tooth repaired. Failure to carry out this program of "preventive dentistry" will lead only to pain from involvement of the nerve tissue and ultimately to removal of the tooth.

The elimination of infection, potential foci of infection, inflammation and pain in the oral region should be part of the patient's course of therapy. The patient's chewing ability should be restored to an acceptable level by replacing missing teeth and restoring decayed teeth. Often the restoration of dentition gives the patient a considerable psychological boost by improving facial form or speech.

Periodontal Disease

This includes a group of diseases affecting the supporting tissues of the teeth. The incidence of these diseases increases with age; also it is considerably greater among the poor than among those in better financial circumstances. The most common of these diseases is gingivitis, which produces minor inflammatory changes in the gum line. Often it may be prevented by regular brushing of the teeth and scaling of the tartar. When, however, the inflammation extends beyond the gum line to the supporting tissues, it may result in breakdown of the alveolar bone and periodontal membrane. The disease is then usually known by the term "pyorrhea." In this condition, the support of the teeth may be seriously damaged, and if the disease continues to progress, loss of teeth will eventually occur. As a matter of fact, in adults, pyorrhea constitutes one of the major causes of loss of teeth. After the age of 35 years,

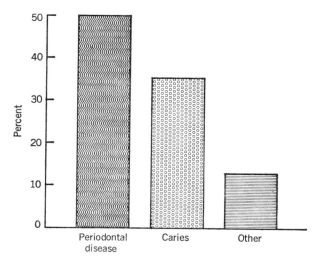

Fig. 27. Tooth loss from periodontal disease, caries, and other causes. (Dentistry in National Health Program, ADA. 1971. Copyright by the American Dental Association. Reprint by permission.)

more teeth are lost from periodontal disease than from dental caries.

Malocclusion

This is a disharmony in the relationship between the upper and lower teeth and may be responsible for many abnormal sequelae, including periodontal disease and speech defects, as well as emotional difficulties as a result of disfigurement. While, at the present time, little can be done to prevent its occurrence, much can be done to prevent its progress, and a great deal may be accomplished in terms of rehabilitation. Patients with malocclusion should be referred to their family dentist or orthodontist for expert care.

Oral Cancer

A word should be said on this subject because neoplasms of the head and neck account for approximately 10% of all malignant disease. Oral cancers often lend themselves to early detection. Yet physicians and dentists who look into thousands of mouths often are not as alert as they should be to early signs of cancer. The use of oral cytologic examination by both physicians and dentists should be increased.

Cleft Palate and Harelip

In cleft palate, there is an opening through the roof of the mouth leading to the floor of the nose. It is commonly associated with harelip in which there is a separation in the normal continuity of the upper lip. Approximately one child of every 800 is born with evidence of this condition. Its importance lies in its interference with normal feeding and with the formation of sounds used in normal speech.

Treatment of this condition is expensive and involves

the services of several specialists, including a dentist. Harelip is normally closed by surgery during the first few months of life. Cleft palate is treated later, by surgery or by a prosthetic appliance.

Dental Public Health Programs

The inclusion of dental services among the programs provided by public health agencies dates back many years. It was recognized early that dental disease was not only one of the most prevalent diseases of mankind, but one which could be readily detected through screening programs. It is still common, however, to find school children whose teeth have been badly neglected. This is often due to lack of motivation on the part of parents, but it may also be due to lack of funds. On the other hand, if everyone in the United States were both motivated and financially able to provide himself with adequate dental care, it is doubtful that the present complement of dental manpower would be equal to the task.

Dental public health programs, then, have concerned themselves with the application of all those services known or believed to produce a reduction of dental disease, as well as with the development of programs aimed at bringing about expeditious provision of dental care for all who need it, irrespective of financial means to pay. Thus, public health agencies have been in the forefront of the drive for fluoridation of public water supplies; they have launched dental health educational programs aimed at improvement of nutrition, reduction in consumption of sweets, regular tooth brushing and visits to the dentist. They have also provided dental screening programs, primarily in schools, and have often made dental care available to those unable to afford private care.

7

While public health services have been traditionally directed toward children, increasing interest in the chronic diseases has caused greater consideration to be given to the dental needs of older persons. Public health dental services for older groups in the population, however, have not been too well developed as yet. Lightweight portable dental equipment is available to permit the dentist to offer the homebound patient a rather complete range of dental services. Some home-care programs employ dental hygienists for prophylaxis and for dental health education.

A program of dental health for children should be comprehensive so as to meet the total dental health needs of every child. The program should include, but not be limited to, the following elements.

Preventive Program. There are available preventive techniques of demonstrated effectiveness for the prevention of dental diseases. These should be employed in their full range, and all dentists should be made aware of the benefits to be realized from their application in communities and to the individual patient.

Fluoridation of Communal Water Supplies. Every program should have the benefit of fluoridation of the communal water supply to reduce dental caries by approximately 60%. When there is no communal water supply, the alternative uses of fluorides should be programmed. State action, when necessary, should be sought to require the fluoridation of all community water supplies. Federal and state support should be provided for all communities in the form of incentives to foster the fluoridation of the water supply. These incentives may take the form of a subsidy for the purchase of equipment and supplies and the employment of personnel for the fluoridation program.

Topical Agents. Where the fluoridation of communal

water supplies is not feasible, provision should be made for the topical application of fluorides, or other anti-cariogenic agents by dentists in private practice or on a public health basis.

Dietary Fluoride Supplements. Provision should be made, when necessary, for the use of dietary fluoride supplements either through public health programs or on the prescription of a physician or dentist.

Anti-Cariogenic Dentifrices. The use of anti-cariogenic dentifrices on a public health or individual basis should be encouraged.

Control of the Consumption of Sweets. Educational campaigns should be conducted to reduce the frequency of consumption of sweets in the diets of all children. Special attention should be given to the elimination of the sale of sweets in schools.

Toothbrushing Instruction. Toothbrushing instruction and oral prophylaxis at regular intervals, starting at 3 years of age, should be encouraged.

Malocclusion. Carious teeth should be restored to maintain normal occlusion, spaces resulting from the early loss of primary teeth should be maintained, and deleterious oral habits should be discouraged.

Patient Education. Provision should be made for a comprehensive and continuing program of patient education in all treatment programs.

Treatment Services. The program should provide all indicated treatment services which are necessary to restore and maintain the dental and total health of the child patient.

Because dental health is directly related to total health and because the oral-facial region is an essential part of everyone's appearance and well-being, the value of oral health should occupy a high priority on the nation's health agenda. As education and income levels rise, the demand for dental services increases.

Prevention should include all proven measures, such as fluoridation of communal water supplies, topical application of fluorides when indicated, oral prophylaxis, plaque control, and effective personal home care.

1. Treatment of congenital anomalies such as cleft palate and lip.
2. Dental health education for new parents (by physician, nurse, well-baby clinics, and so forth) with emphasis on:
   a. prevention of dental caries (good dietary habits, fluoride intake),
   b. prevention of malocclusion (habit control, maintenance of all primary teeth),
   c. prevention of periodontal disease (effective home care methods),
   d. prevention of injuries (appropriate parental surveillance).
3. First visit to dentist should take place soon after all primary teeth have erupted. Some pedodontists recommend that the first visit be made by 18 months of age so parents can be counseled and so the child can become acquainted with the dentist before serious problems have developed. For the 18-month-old child, this appointment would be limited to an examination and appropriate counseling of the parents. For the 30- to 36-month-old child, the first appointment should include:
   a. an oral prophylaxis,
   b. a complete examination (including radiographs),
   c. application of topical caries-preventive agents, if indicated,
   d. counseling of parents on treatment needs and

ways in which the family can prevent the full range of oral diseases through effective home care measures.

4. Treatment appointments should include all measures necessary to eliminate oral disease and prevent the onset of additional problems by:
   a. restoring carious or fractured teeth,
   b. extracting teeth that cannot be restored,
   c. maintaining dental arch size when indicated,
   d. removing all irritants to supporting tissues,
   e. aiding child to eliminate unfavorable oral habits,
   f. correcting malocclusions such as functional crossbites,
   g. reinforcing measures for effective home care by repeated counseling.
5. Dental health maintenance should be scheduled for each child as required, and intervals can vary from 3 months to 12 months. Such visits should include:
   a. an oral prophylaxis,
   b. a complete examination for dental caries, malocclusion, periodontal disease, anomalies, and evidence of trauma,
   c. application of caries-preventive agents, if indicated,
   d. restoration of carious teeth,
   e. repeated counseling about effective home care.
6. Dental health education in the schools should supplement the efforts of the providers of dental services by informing and motivating students accurately and effectively.
   a. Teachers should be prepared adequately in the ways to attain optimum oral health and how to transmit this information effectively to students.

    b. Information on dental health should be transmitted to students at the lowest grade level and continued through the secondary grade levels.

7. Special oral health problems.
    a. Injuries to the oral-facial region are common during the childhood years. Since many dental injuries can be prevented by use of automobile seat belts, a dental emphasis should be included in encouraging their use. Mouth guards should be used by those participating in contact sports to prevent injury. Whenever a dental injury occurs, it should be treated immediately.
    b. Malocclusions occur in about 50% of the population, and 20% have problems that detract from appearance and interfere with chewing and speech. Careful examination, diagnosis, and proper treatment at the optimal time can minimize the problems. A crippling malocclusion can be just as damaging as a crippled limb and can result in serious emotional and social problems.
    c. Dental anomalies such as cleft palate and lip, dysplasia of enamel and dentin, and missing and supernumerary teeth can be disfiguring. Failure to provide effective treatment may result in educational, employment, or social problems.
    d. Sick or handicapped children frequently have dental problems that are neglected for various reasons. This neglect may intensify other problems.

8. Dental care for adults should be uncomplicated and relatively inexpensive for those who reach adulthood in an optimal state of oral health achieved through the program described.

 a. Most adults will develop carious lesions infre-
  quently.
 b. Most adults require special attention to the supporting tissues, for example,
   1. more comprehensive home care,
   2. more comprehensive oral prophylaxis (root
    planing and soft tissue curettage),
   3. elimination of occlusal interferences.
 c. All adults should be examined routinely for oral
  cancer and other pathologic conditions and receive the appropriate treatment.
 d. Missing teeth should be replaced as promptly
  as possible.
 e. Elderly patients, especially the hospitalized or
  homebound, will require special methods to
  maintain their optimum oral health.

The responsibilities for preventing dental disease
through the application of preventive measures can be
divided into three classes:

 those that are automatic and require no deliberate
 action by the individual, for example, oral prophylaxis, topical application of fluoride or fluoridation
 of drinking water;

 those that require positive action on the part of the
 professional provider of services, for example, oral
 prophylaxis, topical application of fluoride, dietary
 counseling, instruction in plaque control and in a
 personal oral hygiene regimen;

 those that require deliberate action and change of
 behavior on the part of the individual after he receives professional advice.

In all three of these areas, much more research is
needed before the full potential for preventing dental
disease will be realized.

Dental Auxiliaries

Recent dental manpower studies have experimented with performance of additional duties by auxiliaries and with the training required to prepare them satisfactorily. In every study, the productivity of dentists has increased by the use of auxiliaries with expanded functions, and the most recent experiment reported that dentists' productivity increased by 130% over the conventional four-handed dentistry arrangement. Teaching dentists to be more productive through the full utilization of auxiliaries appears to be a more practical, economical, and efficient approach to delivering more high quality care to more people.

Although advances in dental technology over the past decade have changed many clinical procedures, the increased use of auxiliaries has been the major factor in increasing the productivity of dentists. The concept of efficient utilization of dental assistants at the chair by dentists is not new, but its widespread adoption has occurred mostly within the past 10 years. This may be the result of programs now in every dental school which teach students how to utilize dental auxiliaries. These programs, also known as four-handed dentistry, were based on earlier studies which demonstrated that the productivity of dentists was increased by about one-third with the addition of one assistant, and by more than two-thirds with the addition of a second assistant.

The dental hygienist is often utilized in one or more of the following ways:

A. As a Clinician.
    She can provide prophylactic care including topical sodium fluoride. She can also be used as a screener, for example, in school health programs.

B. As an Administrator.
   She can organize, staff and program community oral
   health facilities.
C. As an Educator.
   She can instruct health consumers (adults and children) on a one to one or a group basis and help
   motivate persons to change their oral health habits.

The dental hygienist is invaluable in school health
programs, working with teachers to integrate oral
health instruction into the curriculum.

In recent years, another auxiliary, the expanded function dental auxiliary, has emerged on the scene. With
appropriate training and under the supervision of a
dentist, this individual can perform a wide range of
clinical functions previously carried out only by dentists, including the completion of restorations. The exact nature of the functions performed depends upon
state law. This can free dentists to concentrate on more
complex dental tasks and to treat additional patients.
This increased productivity can help alleviate dental
manpower shortages and, hopefully, contain costs.

Quality of Dental Care

No elements of a health care program are more important than quality review and methods of payment.
These administrative issues are crucial to a program's
effectiveness in terms of the improvement of health, the
satisfaction of the consumers and the providers of care,
and the participation of the providers. Because payment systems and provisions for review are also vulnerable to abuse, misunderstanding, and criticism, they
require sound planning and continuing surveillance.

To achieve high quality the program must include:

a. disease prevention,
b. thorough diagnosis of each patient's oral, general and attitudinal statistics,
c. treatment of diseases and correction of defects,
d. maintenance of an optimal level of oral health,
e. maximization of the utilization of services in relation to cost and available resources.

In many ways, the dental audit is simpler than a medical audit. It is not too difficult, for example, to develop statistical data detailing, let's say, the ratio of fillings to extractions.

There are three basic questions to be answered by a dental audit:

1. Is the procedure necessary?
2. Was it done well or properly?
3. Was the patient benefited?

Studies have indicated that the financial barrier is only one of several deterrents to obtaining dental care. This seems to be borne out by relatively low utilization rates under some dental programs with all or most of the cost barriers removed; utilization rates in a few plans have not been substantially higher than the 42% annual utilization of dental services in the general public, and in some programs they have been even lower.

Group Practice

About 71% of the practicing dentists in the United States are engaged in solo practice. The backbone of the dental delivery system is, therefore, the solo practitioner; but there is a trend toward more group practices. The predominant mode of solo practice likely is an outgrowth of the way dentists are taught to practice as students in dental school, where group practice, until recent years, has rarely been mentioned.

The distribution of dental specialists is even more imbalanced than the distribution of general practitioners. Moreover, the roles of the specialists are not clearly defined and, as a consequence, their services are not optimally utilized.

From the experience of those engaged in group practices, there appear to be certain advantages to group practice for both patients and dentists.

For patients, some of the advantages are:

better accessibility of service with more and better use of auxiliary personnel; no long waiting periods, emergency treatment available at all times,

a wider variety of dental personnel and dental equipment available,

group consultation readily available,

built-in quality controls of services rendered,

better utilization of specialists' services.

For dental personnel, some of the advantages are:

group purchase economy,

lower percentage for overhead,

wider range of equipment and auxiliary personnel,

dentist is free of more administrative tasks,

economies in laboratory services, accounting, legal, housekeeping and maintenance services,

opportunities for auxiliary training and advancement,

more security during recovery from illness or accident,

more fringe benefits: vacations, pension plans, insurance coverage,

patients are cared for by dentists in the group during absences.

There is relatively little dental care available at low cost or without cost to the indigent or the medically indigent population, partly because public health and welfare budgets often omit dental care. Most state Medicaid programs include some level of dental benefits, ranging from comprehensive care to emergency services only. Office of Economic Opportunity programs have provided free dental care to many additional persons: for instance, Head Start programs covered 685,000 preschool children in 1970. Other common sources for free or low-cost care are dental school clinics and school health programs. However, many communities have none of these.

Dental Insurance

Except for a few isolated cases, dental insurance on a group basis began as a fringe benefit of employment in 1954 and has expanded in this form. As yet, dental insurance of comparable level is not generally available on an individual basis, nor does it appear that this type of coverage will be widely available in the immediate future. To make individual dental coverage feasible for insurance carriers, it would be necessary to charge substantial premiums and include limitations on benefits and various deterrents to 100% utilization. A likely exclusion would be treatment of pre-existing conditions. The feasibility of individual coverage is diluted by the fact that those individuals who are sufficiently motivated to purchase dental coverage would do so in order to use the insurance; therefore, high utilization could reasonably be expected.

Under most prepaid dental programs, the employer pays the entire premium and the beneficiaries contribute to the cost of their care through deductibles or coinsurance. Annual maximums on benefits are common.

Coverage may vary from basic benefits only to a full range of dental care including orthodontics.

Dental coverage is offered by about 40 dental service plans sponsored by state dental societies, the major private health insurance carriers, and some state or local Blue Cross and Blue Shield plans. Coverage is also provided by various types of prepaid group dental practices employing salaried dentists and through self-insurance arrangements.

By early 1971, more than 10 million persons were estimated to be eligible for dental care under some type of prepayment plan. In the past few years, the population covered by dental insurance has increased substantially from less than a million in 1960 to close to 55 million by 1978 according to estimates made by the American Dental Association. In other words approximately 25% of the population now has some degree of dental insurance.

A complicating factor in dental insurance is that dental disease is irreversible as well as universal. Treatment may be deferred, but postponement will increase and compound the treatment needs. Surveys show that needs for dental care become greater with the passage of time since the last dental visit. Therefore, low utilization in a dental care program may be favorable for controlling present costs but may indicate dental neglect that will eventually result in higher costs when nonusers finally avail themselves of the coverage.

Dental health needs are best met by a program with a high utilization rate, but the insuring agencies have a conflicting perspective. From the standpoint of an insurer's finances, low utilization is desirable; from the standpoint of longterm financial security, high utilization during the first year is often followed by relatively stable costly maintenance needs in successive years.

This conflicting perspective has been referred to as the "utilization-cost dilemma."

Status of Methods of Payment. Most dental care is provided on the traditional fee-for-service basis and is paid for out-of-pocket by the patient. The national dental bill in 1977 was estimated by the U.S. Department of Commerce at approximately $10 billion, or a per capita dental expenditure of $45.11. Based on the finding of the National Health Survey that 42% of the population sees a dentist once a year, the average expenditure per person who saw a dentist in 1970 can be estimated at $49.30.

REFERENCES

A Private Practitioner Looks at Dental Manpower Planning, by W. Kelley Carr, D.D.S. Presented at National Dental Health Conference, March 1973.

Ast, D. B.: Dental Public Health, in Sartwell: *Preventive Medicine and Public Health,* Maxcy and Rosenau (Eds.) 10th Ed., New York, Appleton-Century-Crofts Inc., 1973.

Commission on the Survey of Dentistry in the United States, The Survey of Dentistry, Final Report, American Council on Education, Washington, D.C., 1961.

Dental Experience in Pre-paid Group Practice, by Max H. Schoen, D.D.S. Presented at Conference on H.M.O.s and Dentistry, February 1973.

Dentistry in National Health Programs, American Dental Association, October 1971.

East, B. R.: Relation of Dental Caries in City Children by Sex, Age and Environment, Amer. J. Dis. Children *61*: 494, 1941.

Increased Use of Expanded Function Dental Auxiliaries Would Benefit the Consumer, Dentists and Taxpayers, Report to the Congress by the Comptroller General of the United States, Washington, D.C., 1979.

Ingram, W. T.: A Report, Water Fluoridation Practices in

Major Cities of the United States, The New York State Department of Health, New York University College of Engineering, 1957.

Klein, H.: The Dental Status and Dental Needs of Young Adult Males Rejectable or Acceptable for Military Service according to Selective Service Dental Requirements, Public Health Reports 56:1369, 1941.

Social Security Bulletin, Vol. 41, Washington, D.C., July, 1978.

Quality Review Factors: The Dental Audit, by Jay W. Friedman, D.D.S. Presented at Conference on H.M.O.s and Dentistry, February 1973.

Unpublished paper by Marlene Klyvert, R.D.H. Presented at National Dental Health Conference, Chicago, March 1973.

Chapter 11

Mental Health, Alcoholism
and Drug Addiction

MENTAL HEALTH

Extent of the Problem

It has been estimated that there are approximately
the same number of beds provided in the United States
for the mentally ill as there are for all other ailments
combined. Each year, more than 300,000 persons are
admitted into mental hospitals in the United States.
One and a half million individuals visit clinics and private physicians with problems primarily emotional in
origin. It has further been estimated that approximately
half of all persons visiting private physicians for any
reason have an emotional problem and approximately
one-third of the patients seen at general hospitals have
illnesses which are primarily emotional in origin. It has
been roughly estimated that at any given time approximately 10% of the population of the United States has
some form of emotional disorder which requires treatment.

Among patients hospitalized for mental illness, almost half have schizophrenia. Among other important diagnoses are mental disorders associated with the process of aging, alcoholism and depression. Schizophrenia tends to appear early in life; depression is usually found at middle age, while arteriosclerotic senile psychoses occur during old age. Mental illness appears to be more common among women than men. Alcoholic psychosis is, however, much more frequent in men than in women. Neuroses are seemingly more common than psychoses among the upper socioeconomic group, whereas the reverse is true in the lower socioeconomic group.

Over many years, hundreds of millions of dollars have been expended in the United States for the construction of, or additions to, mental hospitals. Tradi-

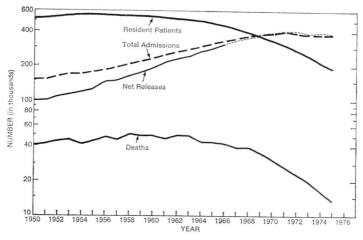

Source: National Institute of Mental Health. June 1977.

Fig. 28. Number of resident patients, total admissions, net releases, and deaths, State and County mental hospitals, United States, 1950-1975.

tionally, patients have been admitted to these institutions, which have been commonly located at a distance from the major population centers, in isolation from the communities in which they have lived, often for many years and, in many cases, for life. Mental illness has had, over the centuries, a stigma which still exists to a considerable extent, although this attitude is changing and, as will be shown later in this chapter, is likely to change further for the better in the future. However, because of the nature of emotional illness, this stigma will probably never disappear entirely.

Recent Trends

While, as has been pointed out above, considerable funds and much effort have been expended in the construction of mental hospital facilities, relatively little, until recently, has been spent on preventive and community-oriented mental health programs. This too is now undergoing considerable change. There has been a marked trend, in recent years, not only to admit more patients to mental hospitals, but also to discharge them more rapidly. The newer drugs used in the treatment of mental disorders undoubtedly have had a marked influence favoring this change.

First admissions to State and County mental hospitals increased from 130,000 in 1962 to 164,000 in 1969 —an increase of 25%—and then declined to a little over 120,000 by 1975. Concurrent with this change, there has been a steady decrease in the resident population of these hospitals, an increase in re-admissions and a decrease in the average length of stay.

In 1962, first admissions age 65 and older constituted 22% of the total, whereas in 1975 these admissions represented less than 7% of the total. On the other hand, first admissions of the age group under 24 years rose from 18% of the total in 1962 to almost 37% in 1975.

Number and per cent distribution of additions to State and County mental hospitals by sex and diagnosis, United States, 1969 and 1973. *Source*: National Institute of Mental Health. Statistical Note 117. June, 1975.

Diagnosis	Both Sexes		Males		Females	
	1969	1973	1969	1973	1969	1973
	Number					
Total, all diagnoses ...	458,918	442,530	265,267	272,619	193,651	169,911
Mental retardation ..	14,146	13,685	8,740	8,341	5,406	5,344
Alcohol disorders	102,051	111,910	85,830	89,076	16,221	22,834
Drug disorders	14,032	25,455	9,754	18,709	4,278	6,746
OBS assoc. with cerebral arteriosclerosis senile brain disease	33,289	20,902	16,521	10,616	16,768	10,286
Other OBS	20,190	13,953	11,995	8,174	7,782	5,779
Schizophrenia	146,121	145,921	69,688	81,098	76,433	64,823
Depressive disorders ..	50,124	46,484	16,298	15,778	34,239	30,706
Other psychoses	9,441	4,334	4,075	1,712	5,366	2,622
Other neuroses	13,290	9,313	5,365	3,267	7,925	6,046
Personality disorders ..	33,962	25,231	23,365	19,528	10,597	5,703
Transient situational disturbances	12,328	13,778	6,582	7,732	5,746	6,046
All other diagnoses ..	9,944	11,564	7,054	8,588	2,890	2,976
	Per cent					
Total, all diagnoses	100.0	100.0	100.0	100.0	100.0	100.0
Mental retardation ...	3.1	3.1	3.3	3.1	2.8	3.1
Alcohol disorders	22.2	25.3	32.4	32.7	8.4	13.4
Drug disorders	3.0	5.8	3.7	6.9	2.2	4.0
OBS assoc. with cerebral arteriosclerosis senile brain disease	7.3	4.7	6.2	3.9	8.7	6.1
Other OBS	4.4	3.1	4.5	3.0	4.0	3.4
Schizophrenia	31.8	33.0	26.3	29.7	39.4	38.2
Depressive disorders ..	10.9	10.5	6.1	5.8	17.6	18.1
Other psychoses	2.1	1.0	1.5	0.6	2.8	1.5
Other neuroses	2.9	2.1	2.0	1.2	4.1	3.6
Personality disorders ..	7.4	5.7	8.8	7.2	5.5	3.4
Transient situational disturbances	2.7	3.1	2.5	2.8	3.0	3.5
All other diagnoses ..	2.2	2.6	2.7	3.1	1.5	1.7

Significant changes have also occurred in the diagnostic composition of admissions. Alcoholic disorders accounted for 25% of admissions in 1973, while schizophrenia represented 33%; brain syndromes decreased from 12% in 1969 to 8% in 1973.

The total number of patients in State and County mental hospitals has been declining for the past 18 years. For the 5 years 1967-1971 the number fell from 426,000 to 308,000. Accompanying this decline, there has been a continued increase in the number of patients released alive from these hospitals. Since 1955, the number has more than tripled. Some of the factors producing this decline include increased availability of alternate care facilities including outpatient and aftercare, and the introduction and expansion of community mental health centers.

In 1939, there were only some 40 general hospitals which maintained facilities and services for psychiatric patients. After World War II, however, this picture began to change, so that by 1954 more than 600 general hospitals were admitting psychiatric patients. In 1961, the report of the Joint Commission on Mental Illness recommended that every general hospital of 100 beds and over have a psychiatric unit. By 1970, there were 766 general hospitals in the United States with separate psychiatric inpatient services.

Manpower resources in mental health are limited while demands are heavy and increasing, and efforts to close the gaps by training programs must be continued.

The Cause of Mental Illness

While epidemiologic studies on the etiologic factors involved in mental illness have been many and varied, much is still unknown concerning the causative factors. When the complexities of genes and chromosomes were first being studied, many tended to believe that heredity was the predominant determinant in a person's character. Today, however, we believe that heredity and environment both play important roles in human growth.

Longitudinal studies of children have clearly demonstrated, however, that irrespective of environmental similarities, children exhibit personality differences at birth and these differences remain.

Mental disorders may be divided into those conditions produced as a result of brain injury and those which occur in apparently healthy individuals. In the latter case, the person appears to behave normally until a certain time, which may be clearly delineated or quite indistinct. After this time, however, behavior changes. The obvious question is what makes it change. Is it something that has suddenly happened or has the change been developing over some period of time? There is a rather large psychiatric school of thought which believes that, in this second category of mental illness, repeated traumatic conditions occurring during life, particularly in the early formative years, may ultimately produce symptoms of mental illness, especially when disturbances are superimposed upon a congenitally weak personality structure. It is this belief that forms the essential ingredient in the development of preventive mental health programs in the United States today.

THE OBJECTIVES OF MENTAL HEALTH PROGRAMS

As Lemkau has stated, the overall goal of mental health is:

1. The prevention of more serious and handicapping illness

2. The removal of sources of stress from family and social environment
3. The making available of services of special personnel to the broader horizons of the mental health program

Prevention

Brain Damage. Major advances have been made in the prevention of mental disease due to brain injury. General paresis due to inadequate treatment of syphilis is now rare among patients admitted to mental hospitals. Pellagra has also disappeared, for practical purposes, as a cause of mental illness in the United States. Among other steps taken to prevent brain damage are adequate prevention against lead poisoning and against a variety of drugs which may produce brain injury.

Personality Development. The basis for the emphasis that is now placed on personality development is the hypothesis that mental disorders are, to a considerable degree, the result of reaction to the stresses of life superimposed upon a genetically determined or early developmental personality weakness. Thus, it is thought that any steps that can be taken to ensure the proper development of personality and to attend at an early date to emotional difficulties that may occur may have an important influence on preventing the development of subsequent serious mental disorders.

Prenatal Care

Studies have indicated that the mother who is emotionally well-adjusted tends to deliver with fewer complications. A prospective mother is concerned during pregnancy, about her capacity for carrying and, subsequently, caring for her child. She is also concerned about relations with her husband during the pregnancy and following delivery. Sometimes the pregnancy is unwanted. In other instances there may be a concern for sibling rivalry. In any case, it is clear that pregnancy is a time during which a prospective mother is subject to a variety of adverse influences. Adequate education of the mother in sexual anatomy and physiology and about the effect of childbirth on her body, the method of delivery, and so forth, can do much to allay anxiety and fears, either imaginary or real. This may, of course, be a routine part of prenatal care in the physician's office. It has also been successfully carried out in community-organized mothers' classes, which are usually developed by the Red Cross or by other health agencies.

Prematurity and Birth Defects

When a baby is born prematurely, the parents may feel that the child is in some way different from others and that he will not develop properly. This feeling is even stronger when the child is born with an obvious defect. The parents commonly blame themselves and have feelings of guilt and unworthiness. Furthermore, this blame may be projected upon the infant, who may become disliked for having brought shame on the parents. Grandparents often contribute to the already strained relationships between the marital partners by holding either the wife or husband as primarily responsible. Thus, the prevention of prematurity and of birth defects may be an important mental health measure. In addition, counselling and, sometimes, psychiatric assistance may be required.

The Baby and Young Child

The first few years of a child's life are important with respect to both physical and personality development. From a time during which he is completely dependent, the infant gradually assumes increasing responsibility for himself. He learns much from his parents and from others in the immediate environment. He requires love, affection and support. He acquires attitudes from his parents and is quick to react or respond to difficulties between them. Problems may result from the young child's feeding habits and in the course of toilet training. It is clear that this can be a difficult period for both mother and father. Anticipatory guidance is commonly called for and should be an essential part of a pediatrician's care. Well-baby clinics organized in many parts of the country by health departments provide pediatric and counselling services for those unable to afford private care.

The School-Age Child

The child now begins to be measured against other children. This may produce satisfaction in the teacher and parent, or it may not. Often the parents expect too much of their child, and when he does not quite measure up to expectations there is disappointment. Often pressure is applied to mold the child into something close to what the parents want. This may have an adverse effect upon a child who simply cannot do all that is expected of him. Behavior problems among children of school age are common. It has been roughly estimated that approximately 10% of school children have an emotional problem that requires assistance. Counselling of the parents and child may be important. If the emotional disturbance becomes more severe, referral for more expert child guidance may be required.

There has been considerable effort to include within the school curriculum material aimed at promoting mental health. There is, of course, no clear evidence that this is effective in reducing behavior disorders.

Adolescents and Adults

While the early years of life would appear to be those at which most emphasis must be placed in an attempt to prevent serious mental disorders from occurring later in life, counselling and guidance are also desirable in later years. For example, adolescence is a time of great changes in the human body and also a time when emotional difficulties may occur. The time immediately before marriage and during the early years of marriage may also constitute periods of stress, when marital counselling may be of considerable value. Assistance in adapting a worker to a new job or a geriatric patient to a change of occupation necessitated by his physical condition may also be warranted. In all cases, the private physician has an important role to play.

Juvenile Delinquency

The prevention of juvenile delinquency is as much a social as it is a medical problem. Most delinquent children are genetically and physically normal children who have become delinquent because of emotional and environmental stresses with which they are unable to cope. More than half come from broken homes. When the parents do live together, there is often serious discord in the home. There is frequently lack of parental supervision, housing conditions may be poor, and there may be poverty. While many delinquents tend to come from overcrowded sections and pockets of poverty, delinquency is not by any means limited to the lower socioeconomic strata. It occurs to a considerable extent among wealthy families. Sometimes the child may have a physical defect which may have contributed to his problem or he may be mentally retarded.

The primary responsibility for improvements rests with the parents. It is essential, however, for the community to play its part by providing supervised recreational facilities and by giving the children a community responsibility which may help them to feel that they are a part of the community and can play a role in promoting its welfare. In addition to the parents and the community, there is no question that the school, the church and the family physician all have an important part to play. The latter can contribute to the prevention of physical defects; he can provide counselling and can ensure appropriate referral for more expert attention as soon as more serious difficulties appear.

The Community Mental Health Program

The historical background of the mental health movement, based upon hospitalization of those with mental disorders in large isolated public institutions, has already been mentioned. In recent years, however, there has been a trend toward the development of mental health facilities more closely related to the community. Among some of the facilities developed are out-patient clinics for both children and adults, some residential care facilities, consultation services to schools, courts, and welfare and other social agencies. Also there has been increasing acceptance of mentally disturbed patients in general hospitals.

A milestone in the development of community mental health services in the United States was reached in 1961, with the report of the Joint Commission on Mental Illness and Health. Partially as a result of the stimulus arising out of this report, there has been a marked emphasis on the development of mental health programs with a strong community orientation. Basic to this new program is the concept that the old traditional methods of treating patients with mental disease in large public institutions is outmoded, and that these institutions should be substantially reduced in size. Also essential to the development of this newly emerging concept is the establishment of a closer relationship between these public mental hospitals and the communities that they serve.

The important elements of this community mental health program are:

1. Flexibility in the handling of patients with emotional disorders so that they may receive the type of care needed at any particular time with a built-in mechanism for ensuring easy transfer from one type of service to another as, for example, between outpatient clinic and residential care.
2. The provision for continuity of care.
3. Emphasis upon providing services for the patient as close to the patient's home as possible. Every patient should have access to a community mental health center in which there should be provided a wide array of services to all kinds of patients, in all age groups.
4. Emphasis on early intensive treatment and rehabilitation with return of the patient to his family and community as soon as possible.

Under this program, it might well be considered that long-term custodial care is an admission of failure in the treatment program.

The basic components of a community mental health program include:

1. early case finding
2. diagnosis and treatment of mental and emotional disorders at all stages of development
3. rehabilitation services to reduce the disability associated with these disorders

4. consultation services to other health, educational, and welfare agencies
5. in-service training for staff of these agencies
6. mental health education of the public
7. primary preventive and promotional programs to locate and reduce sources of mental and emotional disturbances
8. applied research.

Characteristics of Community Mental Health Centers

1. *Geographic responsibilities*
   Every center provides its services to a catchment area ranging in size from 75,000–200,000 people.
2. *Comprehensive Programs*
   a. Emergency services 24 hours a day.
   b. Consultation and education programs.
   c. Outpatient services.
   d. Inpatient services.
   e. Partial hospitalization (*e.g.,* day care).
3. *Accessibility*
   Must be readily accessible to residents of catchment area.
4. *Continuity of Care*
5. *Responsiveness to Community Needs*
6. *A System of Services*
   Services may not necessarily be housed in one building but may result from an affiliation of several programs working together and coordinated.

Services should be provided for children, adolescents, adults, geriatric patients, alcoholics and drug addicts. A variety of rehabilitation services should be included, with vocational training and recreational therapy available.

The community mental health center should provide

a major resource for both private physicians and psychiatrists. It should also, wherever possible, be affiliated with teaching institutions so that it may serve as a center for training and research.

As of October 1, 1978, 624 community mental health centers were in operation. Their costs are borne by a varying proportion of Federal, state and local funds including fees for services.

Some catchment areas which may encompass more than one jurisdiction have found it difficult to properly coordinate services throughout the area and unnecessary duplication has often occurred. In some others, the geographic area covered is so large that efficient service delivery has proven difficult. There have also been problems in relation to state mental hospitals participation in relation to pre-admission screening and interagency referrals. Finally third-party reimbursement will need to be included if these centers are to remain financially viable.

ALCOHOLISM

Alcoholism constitutes an important public health problem in the United States today. While some consider it a disease, others believe it to be merely a symptom of deeper underlying emotional disorder. The American Medical Association describes alcoholics as "those excessive drinkers whose dependence on alcohol has attained such a degree that it shows a noticeable disturbance or interference with their bodily or mental health, their interpersonal reactions, and their satisfactory social and economic functioning." The National Council on Alcoholism estimates that there are some 70,000,000 people in the United States who drink alcoholic beverages. Most drink socially, but approximately 5,000,000 of these are considered alcoholics. Alcoholism afflicts both men and women of all ages and from all walks of life. Alcoholism also constitutes an important factor in the admission of patients to mental hospitals; many such institutions count a diagnosis of alcoholism as second only to schizophrenia in patients admitted to those facilities. In many mental hospitals, approximately a quarter of all new admissions are for alcoholism. Furthermore, alcoholism not only may produce disability and even death in the patient but also carries with it profound social and economic considerations, often leading to breakdown of the family unit, loss of work and economic deprivation. The problem is made even more intense by the difficulties and uncertainties

Consumption trends for men and women, 1971-1976. *Source*: National Institute on Alcohol Abuse and Alcoholism, Contract ADM 281-76-0020, Washington, D.C., July, 1977.

Type of Drinker	*Percentage in Each Drinking Category*						
	1971	1972	1973	1973	1974	1975	1976
Men							
Abstainer	30	28	25	26	24	27	26
Light	29	29	24	29	24	27	33
Moderate	26	28	29	26	34	26	24
Heavier	15	15	22	19	18	20	18°
(N)	(1084)	(767)	(783)	(783)	(776)	(505)	(1230)
Women							
Abstainer	42	44	42	47	42	45	39
Light	40	34	35	32	32	35	44
Moderate	13	18	17	17	21	15	15
Heavier	5	4	6	4	5	4	3
(N)	(1111)	(770)	(796)	(821)	(803)	(566)	(1340)

°Statistically significant linear trend ($p<.05$), indicating an increase.

Alcohol consumption for males in five age groups, 1971-1976.[a] *Source*: National Institute on Alcohol Abuse and Alcoholism, Contract ADM 281-76-0020, Washington, D.C., July, 1977.

Age[a] Group	Percentage For Each Year							Six Year Average
	1971	1972	1973	1973	1974	1975	1976	
18–20								
Drinkers	77	78	86	77	78	b	82	80
Heavier drinkers	18	22	31	18	28	b	20	24
(N)	(85)	(58)	(71)	(67)	(66)		(104)	
21–34								
Drinkers	84	88	85	84	86	89	85	86
Heavier drinkers	20	17	26	20	21	28	21	22
(N)	(280)	(241)	(268)	(230)	(226)	(163)	(401)	
35–49								
Drinkers	73	76	78	82	80	75	75	77
Heavier drinkers	18	19	25	22	21	20	19	21
(N)	(231)	(174)	(161)	(207)	(210)	(125)	(293)	
50–64								
Drinkers	65	64	68	65	72	67	69	67
Heavier drinkers	16	13	14	20	15	21	22	17
(N)	(234)	(165)	(157)	(166)	(168)	(114)	(256)	
65 and Over								
Drinkers	54	45	46	53	54	36	51	48
Heavier drinkers	6	6	14	12	5	6	2	7
(N)	(252)	(126)	(122)	(106)	(101)		(68)	(175)

[a]No significant linear trends
[b]Insufficient data

involved in treatment. Many alcoholics are not motivated to seek assistance until they are at "rock bottom." Others are helped temporarily, only to return to alcohol after a short time. Alcoholism further constitutes an important complicating factor in the management of coexisting diseases. For example, the treatment of tuberculous patients would be much easier if many were not alcoholics. Superintendents of tuberculosis sanatoria are familiar with the problems of the alcoholic who leaves the hospital against advice primarily to get his drink.

Some Characteristics of the Alcoholic

Denial—The alcoholic fails to recognize his drinking as a problem.

Impulsiveness—He does things on the spur of the moment.

Evasion—He hides his drinking.

Projection—He protects himself by blaming his problem on other people.

Low Frustration Tolerance—Little things upset him.

Helplessness—He feels that every effort to do something about his situation has been to no avail.

Ambivalence—He is torn between stopping drinking and getting another bottle.

Unworthiness—He feels he does not deserve the attention given him.

Manipulation—He is expert at manipulating people and situations to his advantage.

Rationalization—He will commonly say, "I can drink or leave it alone."

Dependence—He often makes great demands on people.

Low Self-esteem—Even though this is often masked by an apparent air of confidence, hostility, he is seething with anger.

The alcoholic usually starts as a "social drinker," but the line between the social drinker and the full-blown alcoholic is often obscure and, in time, is passed when the individual begins to rely upon alcohol as a crutch.

Drinking may begin early in the morning and occur often throughout the day, or there may be periods of abstinence when heavy drinking occurs only after working hours or on weekends or holidays; however, when such bouts do occur, they are uncontrolled and pathologic. The alcoholic exhibits gross behavior disorders, hangovers, loss of control and finally develops alibis, loses his job, his friends and often his wife and family. Many alcoholics develop delirium tremens and convulsions and often go into an almost continuous drunken stupor with brain deterioration and, in some cases, death.

It should be clearly understood that alcoholism is common in all walks of life and is not, in particular, a disease of the poor. As a matter of fact, it tends to be more prevalent in the United States than in many other countries of the world. This may be partially due to higher general income, which enables residents of this country to purchase more alcohol. It is also quite common for a psychotic individual to present as an alco-

Per Cent of Adults Who Drink, by Years of Education, United States, 1963. Mulford, *ibid.*

Years of Education	Per Cent Drinkers
0–7	46
8	60
9–11	70
12	79
13–15	76
16	89
Over 16	79
Total Sample	71%

8

Per Cent of Adults Who Drink, by Occupational Classification, United States, 1963. Mulford, *ibid.*

Occupational Classification	Per Cent Drinkers
laborers	69
farmers, carpenters, painters	67
mechanics, cabinetmakers	76
machinists, salesmen, managers	73
electricians, foremen, nurses	83
musicians, bookkeepers	76
real estate, insurance agents, secretaries	84
buyers, store department heads, veterinarians	80
college professors, scientists, engineers	87
dentists, lawyers, judges, physicians	100

holic. This is true with both schizophrenia and manic-depression. In other cases, alcoholism seems to constitute a method of escape from the individual's inability to face what, in his mind, is a difficult or impossible situation.

Mention must be made here of another serious impact of alcoholism upon community life, namely, the problem of the drinking driver. As is well known, alcoholism is involved in a major proportion of automobile accidents.

Investigations indicate that driving potential is impaired even at low blood alcohol levels. In studies of traffic accidents, information appears to show more than a chance relationship to alcohol consumption. Accidents following drinking are more likely to occur at night and on weekends and to be more severe.

Measures to control the drinking and driving problem have involved three principal approaches.

1. Legislation to prohibit driving while under the influence of alcohol.
2. Laws which provide for punishment of people who violate these laws.
3. Teaching young people to fear the use of alcohol in relation to driving.

Excessive drinking is listed as a contributing factor in more than 20% of divorce cases. Three-quarters of the police efforts are expended in dealing with drinking problems.

A review of the case load of a public health nursing program of most health departments would reveal a substantial number of families in whom at least part of the problem relates to chronic alcoholism in at least one of the family members. For example, where children with physical or emotional problems are continually reported to unresponsive parents, the public health nurse will often find that this neglect can be traced to an alcoholic parent. Public health workers have great difficulty coping with the tuberculous patient who is also an alcoholic.

Control Measures

There appears to be no way of detecting which individual is likely to develop alcoholism, and there appears to be no definite method available at this time for the primary prevention of alcoholism. Therefore, most of the emphasis on controlling the problem has to relate to the handling of the chronic alcoholic. Hopefully, this can begin at an early stage in the patient's alcoholic history; treatment is therefore designed to prevent social, physiologic and psychologic deterioration.

Alcoholics Anonymous was organized in 1935. It is "a fellowship of men and women who share their experience, strength and hope with each other that they may solve their common problem and help others to recover from alcoholism." The only requirement for membership is an honest desire on the part of the applicant to stop drinking. There are more than 5,000 A.A. groups throughout the world, and they have played a major, in fact undoubtedly the largest, role in assisting recovery of alcoholics. The alcoholic cannot control his drinking; he must abstain completely or his alcoholism will become progressively worse. Alcoholics Anonymous provides hope for the individual and a means of facing reality with group interaction and support. It is a spiritually oriented organization, based on reliance on a Higher Power for support.

Apart from the important contribution made by Alcoholics Anonymous, it is clear that the problem of alcoholism requires a medical as well as a social approach. A number of communities have established alcoholic rehabilitation programs with particular emphasis upon psychiatric care, with counselling and associated medical treatment as required. Antabuse is used rather widely as an adjunct to therapy. This drug produces nausea and vomiting when a person drinks alcohol. However, there is little question that psychiatric treatment, including the use of drugs, is not enough. It is essential that other aspects of the alcoholics' problems must be explored, including social, economic, vocational and family problems, and that nothing short of total rehabilitation using all available community resources should be sought. While the private physician should play an important part in rehabilitation of the alcoholic, it is difficult, if not impossible, for him to achieve the desired goal unless he uses the other community resources available. On the other hand, even physicians often look upon the alcoholic as a socially undesirable individual who has not been able to fit into society and who is unwilling to help himself. It is essential that physicians face the problem honestly and endeavor to be of assistance.

Industry, too, has an important responsibility for coping with the alcoholic problem, since it has been estimated that as many as 50% of all alcoholics are employed at all levels, professional, skilled and unskilled. As a matter of fact, management has, in many instances, realized that when it has spent both time and money on training employees, it can ill afford for that employee to deteriorate to the point where he will no longer be of value. Accordingly, some industries have rather well-developed programs designed to assist their alcoholic employees.

Since World War II, with leadership and assistance from the National Council on Alcoholism, information and referral centers have been established in many communities. These are particularly important in areas where alcoholism control activities are conducted on a fragmented and isolated basis.

Insofar as the community is concerned, there is little question that the traditional attitude of local and state governmental agencies toward the alcoholic has not been all it should. Often the alcoholic is picked up and hauled off to jail or to a mental hospital and left to "dry out." On leaving this facility the patient immediately returns to his former habits. There results what may be called the "revolving door," whereby the alcoholic continually travels between the jail and the community, often for years, with no effort on the part of anyone to assist his rehabilitation into the community. Hopefully, this attitude will undergo change, and there will be recognition of the need for bringing total community resources to bear in an attempt to rehabilitate the alcoholic.

Public health nurses can provide many basic services in Community Alcoholism programs. Their work with families places them in a position to identify potential alcoholics and, therefore, they are an important source of case finding and referral activities. Once the alcoholic is brought to treatment, the public health nurse can provide follow-up services and be an effective member of the treatment team.

Alcoholic rehabilitation is also an essential part of the community mental health center program. Therefore, this program must provide the same array of services as it does for other persons with mental disorders. There must be services to assist the alcoholic at home, in outpatient clinics, and in day and night centers; residential treatment and social, vocational, recreational and economic assistance must be made available. Halfway houses are also needed for the alcoholic, where he can mix freely in a suitable environment with others who have similar problems.

Considerable efforts have been placed during the past few years on developing a variety of community programs aimed at rehabilitation of the alcoholic. These programs appear to be much needed.

DRUG ADDICTION

The drug addict is usually looked upon as a misfit and a criminal. In fact, the very act of obtaining the drug necessary to satisfy the addict's craving is a felony. In terms of numbers of people involved, it is difficult to measure the extent of the problem because accurate figures on the number of drug addicts are extremely difficult to secure. While, for example, the National Institute on Drug Abuse estimates that 14,600 drug addicts are located in the District of Columbia, there is little question this is not accurate. It has been roughly estimated that there are more than 500,000 heroin addicts throughout the United States, and this number is certainly subject to considerable revision.

In this country, drug addiction is synonymous with heroin addiction. Marihuana is often used as a step on the road to the use of heroin, while cocaine is of relative unimportance. Heroin is usually taken intravenously because of its almost immediate action. The patient acquires an increasing tolerance so that larger and larger doses must be taken in order to achieve the desired effect. Much of the heroin smuggled into this country is from eastern countries. Once here, it is diluted to a considerable extent and, even in this diluted form, brings high prices.

Drug addiction in the United States is found particularly in major cities and is located mainly in low socioeconomic areas. These same areas have high rates of delinquency and venereal disease. It would seem that the typical drug addict is an individual who is psychologically susceptible and placed in an environment which subjects him to conditions which finally result in his taking drugs. This is particularly true when he associates with a group of friends who are already using narcotics.

Traditionally, youth is a time for experimentation, and to some the forbidden has a special allure. Some young people, therefore, are induced by "friends" to try drugs. Others, however, do so to escape personal anxiety and frustration or the poverty of their surroundings.

Until fairly recent times, cases of drug dependence were uncommon in Great Britain. However, this situation has changed. There has been a marked increase in drug addiction, particularly among adolescents.

Outbreaks of infectious hepatitis are fairly common among heroin addicts, due mostly to their tendency to share syringes with other addicts.

The drug addiction problem is somewhat different for different cultural groups. The middle class amphetamine addict will need to be treated differently from a low income inner city heroin user. Drug addiction and crime are inexorably intertwined. For example, it will cost a heroin addict some $85 to $100 to buy his day's supply of heroin. Turning to crime is the only way he has of getting that much money. Once "hooked," obtaining a continued supply of his drug becomes the main goal of his life. Statistics appear to indicate that the heroin addict's life may be shortened by some 15 to 20 years. The total number of drug addict-related deaths in the country in 1972 was 3,358 of whom almost 6% were teenagers; more than 1,400 deaths occurred in the New York area alone.

DRUGS PRODUCING DEPENDENCY

1. Volatile anesthetic solvents
   e.g. Benzene, gasoline, paint thinner, glue. These agents are sniffed.
2. Hypnotics
   e.g. Barbiturates.
3. Tranquilizers
   e.g. Meprobamate.
4. Narcotic analgesics
   e.g. Opium and its derivatives.
5. Stimulants
   e.g. The amphetamines, cocaine.
6. Hallucinogens
   e.g. LSD.
7. Marihuana

Drugs induce mood changes; at first a feeling of well being, but subsequently less desirable effects such as drowsiness, confusion, irritability and even fear.

The drug addict develops tolerance, that is, increasing amounts of the drug are necessary to obtain the same effect. He also develops physical dependence whereby continued use of the drug is necessary in order for him not to develop withdrawal symptoms. The full-blown heroin addict exhibits dependency, passivity, narcissism, low frustration tolerance, suspiciousness, a disregard of time and irresponsibility.

The effect of the drug is to create a sensation of freedom from worry and pleasant relaxation. Eventually the drug becomes the solution to all of the addict's problems, and he comes to rely on it totally. The cost of acquiring heroin is such as to induce the addict to steal and to resort to other crimes. Ultimately, the addict becomes so totally dependent upon the drug that he may become almost completely bedridden except for the times when he is required to make the effort necessary to secure additional supplies.

If the drug is suddenly withdrawn, the patient experiences what is known as "cold turkey" with serious symptoms, including perspiration, vomiting, diarrhea, and elevation of temperature and pulse rate; these symptoms may lead to death. However, gradual withdrawal of the drug, a method of treatment often used in Great Britain, produces less intense symptoms which somewhat resemble those of a cold.

Control Measures

The treatment of drug addicts has, in general, been marked by repeated failures. The adage, "once a drug addict always a drug addict," has unfortunately been found to be reasonably accurate. Treatment of drug addicts at the two United States Public Health Service hospitals at Fort Worth, Texas, and Lexington, Kentucky, has not been particularly successful in assuring that those discharged remain free of the need for drugs. Possibly, lack of follow-up in the community may account for this. Certainly, no easy solution to this problem has been found yet. It would seem essential, however, that irrespective of the system of treatment, it must include adequate attention to the social, vocational and economic problems besetting the addict, much as in the case of the alcoholic.

Facilities for drug addicts must include:

> inpatient facilities for withdrawal,
> outpatient care,
> halfway houses,
> emergency care 24 hours a day,
> consultation, and
> education services.

It has been demonstrated that making available community resources to the addict is no assurance that he will use them particularly those involving sustained counselling. Furthermore, while it may be possible to assist the addict in locating employment, he seldom stays on the job for more than a few weeks, usually because of his relapse to the use of drugs.

One of the more recent efforts to get known heroin addicts to relinquish the use of that drug involves the use of methadone. Addicts have been maintained on methadone (which is inexpensive) by daily doses administered at a community clinic. It should be noted, however, that addiction to methadone may also occur. Heroin produces severe withdrawal symptoms which are usually over in about 72 hours; withdrawal symptoms from methadone are milder but last well over a week. It is clear that while methadone has been found useful in the treatment of heroin addicts, it is more difficult to "kick" a methadone habit than heroin in the sense that it takes longer, something on the order of 6 months.

REFERENCES

A report on a five-year community experiment of the New York Demonstration. NIMH, U.S. Department of HEW, May, 1963.

Action for Mental Health, Joint Commission on Mental Illness and Health, Final Report, New York, 1961.

Bovet, L.: *Psychiatric Aspects of Juvenile Delinquency,* Geneva, World Health Organization, 1951.

Caplan, G.: *An Approach to Community Mental Health,* New York, Grune & Stratton, Inc., 1961.

——————: *Principles of Preventive Psychiatry,* New York, Basic Books, Inc., 1964.

Drugs of Abuse by Samuel Irwin, Ph.D., University of Oregon Medical School. Guide to Community Control of Alcoholism, APHA, 1968.

Jellinek, E. M.: *The Disease Concept of Alcoholism,* New Haven, Conn., Hillhouse Press, 1960.

Legislative and Administrative Changes Needed in Community Mental Health Centers Program, Report to the Congress by the Comptroller General of the United States, 1979.

Lemkau, P.: *Mental Hygiene in Public Health,* 2nd Ed., New York, McGraw-Hill Book Co., Inc., 1955.

——————: Community planning for mental health, Pub. Health Rep. 76:489, 1961.

Manual on Alcoholism, Committee on Alcoholism of the Council on Mental Health, American Medical Association, Chicago, 1962.

Memo to Director, Division of Research, National Institute on Drug Abuse, February 2, 1978.

Mental Health Centers in the United States—An Overview—S. Feldman and H. H. Goldstein, NIMH, 1971.

Project Dawn 6, National Institute on Drug Abuse, Washington, D.C., 1978.

Psychiatric Services in General Hospitals 1969-1970—National Institute of Mental Health, 1972.

Report on Narcotic Addiction, Council on Mental Health of the American Medical Assn., J.A.M.A., 1957.

Statistical Note 55, NIMH, May, 1971.

Statistical Note 60, NIMH, January, 1972.

Chapter 12

Mental Retardation

Extent of the Problem

The magnitude of the mental deficiency problem can be gleaned from the estimate that some 3% of all infants born will, at sometime during their lives, be regarded as mentally retarded. The nation's mentally retarded number approximately 6 million. Some 200,000 are institutionalized. The etiological factor in 75% of those with mental retardation is unknown. There are, of course, all degrees of the problem, varying from the profoundly retarded who have an extremely low IQ, to the mildly retarded whose IQ may vary between 50 and 70. According to the classification commonly used today, the retarded may be divided into the following three groups according to IQ:

Mildly retarded   IQ 50–70 (about 80–85% of total)
Moderately retarded IQ 35–50 (about 10–15% of total)
Severely retarded IQ less than 35 (about 3–5% of total)

Another useful classification is used in relation to educational programs. A mentally retarded child may be described as *educable,* in which case he may be able to receive some schooling; these children usually have an IQ of between 50 and 75. A *trainable* child is one who may be able to reach a reasonable level of self-care and economic usefulness; his IQ usually ranges from 25 to 50. A child who is *totally dependent* is one who requires assistance in even routine matters and who usually has to be institutionalized, probably for life.

The magnitude of the problem of mental retardation has also changed to a considerable extent as a result of improvements in the treatment of disease. Before the advent of antibiotics, large numbers of mentally retarded children, particularly those severely retarded, died in institutions before becoming adults. Death was commonly due to infection for which there was no effective treatment. Today, with modern therapeutic methods available, these severely retarded children commonly live not only to adulthood, but into middle and old age. This has become even more pronounced with other improvements in medical technology which have changed the prognosis for mental defectives who have associated medical conditions, such as severe heart disease.

Thus, the number of mentally retarded in institutions is increasing and, today, one finds considerable numbers of older persons living in such facilities.

The Cause of Mental Deficiency

More than 200 causes of mental retardation have been identified. These include influences affecting the central nervous system prior to birth and those which affect its functioning after birth. The cause of mental retardation is unknown, in many cases, whereas in others there are obvious organic defects or disease entities which are recognizable as the etiologic factor involved. This is also true, of course, with trauma. One area of considerable study relates to the viral infections, such as rubella, occurring during pregnancy, particularly in the first trimester. There is some evidence that a number of viral infections occurring during this period may lead to mental retardation in the unborn child. Certain metabolic disorders in the mother, such as hypothyroidism, may also lead to mental deficiency in the child if treatment is not given during pregnancy. Care should be taken when drugs are prescribed during pregnancy, particularly in the early months, since there have been instances where the administration of certain drugs has appeared to lead to the development of abnormalities in the fetus. Chromosomal studies have revealed association of chromosome disorders with certain types of mental retardation, such as Down's syndrome. This has important implications for genetic counselling. Complications of pregnancy, such as toxemia or hemorrhage, are also often associated with development of mental retardation in the infant. This is particularly true if the infant is born prematurely.

Phenylketonuria is important in relationship to the subsequent development of mental retardation in the child. Its importance is emphasized by the fact that retardation may be essentially prevented by appropriate dietary management. Cretinism is another instance in which early diagnosis may be particularly important. Among the infections, meningitis and encephalitis often result in mental retardation.

Importance of Early Recognition

The child with mental retardation frequently exhibits slowness in locomotion, coordination, speech, and other forms of activity at an early date. Unfortunately, however, parents, through either ignorance or unwillingness to accept the inevitable, often do not seek advice at this early stage. On the other hand, other parents spend many months going from door to door, visiting a variety of physicians, psychologists and others in the hope that they will be told that their child is not retarded. Part of their resistance to accepting a diagnosis of mental retardation is also due to a feeling of shame and to the fact that they blame themselves for the defect. Early recognition and definitive diagnosis are important for the child and for the rest of the family, both in terms of ensuring early family acceptance of the circumstances and because planning for the child's future should start as early as possible. Further, the child may have associated medical conditions which require treatment.

On the other hand, early diagnosis is not always a simple matter; often the family physician may need assistance from other health personnel, such as the psychologist, psychiatrist or pediatrician, before a certain diagnosis can be obtained.

Another important reason for establishing early diagnosis is that some forms of retardation are preventable, *e.g.*, that associated with phenylketonuria. Certainly, in all cases where an infant is slow to grasp objects, to hold up his head, sit, walk and talk, or if he does not appear to respond, the physician should investigate further.

Prevention of Retardation

While it is true that today's knowledge does not permit the prevention of most mental deficiencies, many opportunities are available. For example, purposeful exposure of little girls to rubella may serve to avoid subsequent development of the disease during pregnancy, when it might lead to retardation in the infant.

Similarly, early detection of phenylalanine in the blood of a newborn infant will enable development of retardation to be avoided by placing the child on a low phenylalanine diet. The use of seat belts in automobiles may reduce brain damage from head trauma, while early thorough treatment of erythroblastosis may prevent kernicterus. Good prenatal care may help reduce prematurity and complications during pregnancy. Genetic counselling should play an important role in reducing the incidence of mental deficiency. In this connection, family planning programs may be appropriate.

Other preventive steps include early diagnosis and treatment of syphilis in the pregnant woman, avoidance of x-ray study during the first trimester and thorough treatment of maternal diabetes. Care to be taken during the delivery includes avoidance of excessive anesthesia and cesarean section, whenever possible.

Management of the Mentally Defective Child

The earliest problem with which the physician is confronted when a diagnosis of retardation in a child is made is that of dealing with the reaction of the parents. Often the parents do not believe the diagnosis; frequently they develop guilt feelings, blaming themselves, and in some cases somebody else, such as the physician who delivered the baby. Counselling of the parents is therefore extremely important. The parents will need to accept the fact that their child is retarded and that his intellectual development will be limited. The parents will need to cooperate with the physician if the future management of the child is to be successful. Relationships of the retarded child with others in the family will have to be discussed, and they, too, will have to understand and learn to live with the situation.

This is, indeed, a difficult time for the parents. The

wise physician will devote considerable time and effort to creating a favorable climate in order for the retarded child to be properly accepted in the family group. Without attention to this one problem, many of the efforts spent in assisting the child in his future years may be wasted.

It should be understood that many professional disciplines will need to play a role in the management of the retarded child. Associated medical defects may require the services of medical or surgical specialists. The psychiatrist or psychologist will often be needed; the social worker, special teacher and vocational counsellor will all have a part to play. Speech therapy and specialized dental care are frequent requirements.

Parents must understand that the child's development will be slow, often painfully so. Educable children can be taught in special classes, where they are available. Trainable children can, with expert guidance, learn useful skills. Where day-care centers are available these can afford welcome relief for the overburdened mother and at the same time provide the child with an opportunity to associate with others similar to himself. Emphasis must be placed on making the retarded individual as self-sufficient as possible, and he should be trained for work for which he is equipped.

A high proportion of mentally retarded persons have associated health defects. This is particularly so in the severely retarded. Common problems include hearing and speech defects, impairment of vision and seizures; neuromuscular disorders are frequent, as are emotional problems. Thus, it is essential in working with the mentally retarded to recognize and to manage these associated difficulties properly.

Community Services for the Retarded

Even today, community services for the mentally retarded are in short supply. In too many states, most severely retarded individuals either spend most of their lives in large, often overcrowded, institutions, or they eke out an existence at home with little outside help available. Furthermore, in many institutions for the mentally defective, the program content leaves much to be desired and often provides only limited means for training residents for semi-independent living outside of the institution. Fortunately, however, considerable interest is currently being engendered in developing a more active program at the community level. Community programs must include consideration of the development of a variety of facilities, now either nonexistent or in short supply. This includes the establishment of comprehensive diagnostic clinics and the initiation of programs aimed at prevention of unnecessary retardation, for example, community-wide detection of phenylketonuria (PKU). It also includes the establishment of day-care centers with well-rounded counselling and activity programs, together with the establishment of sufficient classes in the public schools, so that special teaching facilities may be made available to the retarded. Both short-term and long-term residential facilities more closely related to the community must be developed. These should have active recreational and vocational programs, with emphasis on training of the retarded for useful occupations and some degree of independence. Plans must include the development of workshops for the retarded and a close working relationship with industry, aimed at motivating management to employ mentally retarded persons. In this connection, it has been found that retarded individuals, specially trained for a specific job, can operate as effectively as a normal person and, in some cases, even more so.

An adequate community program will also include provision for retarded children of preschool age, including day-care centers for this age group, extensive recreational programs specially designed for retarded persons, and a variety of group activities.

Obviously, one of the great problems that must be met by our educational institutions is that of manpower development and training. Clearly, many disciplines must receive special training in the problems of the mentally retarded if they are to play their roles. It will also be necessary to do much to motivate persons to devote part or all of their professional lives to working with the mentally retarded.

REFERENCES

Mental Retardation, Activities of the U.S. Department of Health, Education and Welfare, July, 1963.

Mental Retardation—*A Handbook for the Primary Physician,* A Report of the A.M.A. Conference on Mental Retardation, April 9-11, 1964.

Pearson, P. H., and Menefee, A. R.: Medical and Social Management of the Mentally Retarded, *GP*, February, 1965.

Chapter 13

Occupational Health

Some 68,000,000 people constitute the working force of the United States. While they are, in many cases, exposed during part or all of the working day to diseases and accidents related directly to their occupations, they are also subject to exactly the same illnesses, not directly related to their occupations, as is the population as a whole. Thus, studies of absenteeism have shown that over 90% of days away from work are due to non-occupational illness and accidents. Currently, approximately 6 work days per person per year are lost as a result of illness or injury. Respiratory ailments are by far the commonest cause of sickness-absenteeism, followed by disorders of the digestive system and other infections. In the chronic diseases, cardiac conditions, disorders of the digestive system, and mental and nervous conditions are among the commonest causes of absenteeism from work.

Lost time from work is important, to both employee and management. To the former it may represent loss of income, while to the latter it may mean loss of production and, in some cases, additional costs incurred as a result of temporary replacement of the absent worker plus the expense of sick-benefit payments.

This chapter is concerned primarily with those conditions more or less directly associated with occupation. Over the years, death and disability from occupational illness and injury have been greatly reduced by industrial health and safety programs.

OCCUPATIONAL DISEASES

Occupational diseases may be divided into three major groups, based upon etiologic factors: those due to chemical agents, those due to physical agents and those due to infections.

Chemical Agents

Dusts. Dusts are finely divided solid particles produced by disintegration of solid materials; they result from processes such as crushing or grinding. Among the most important dusts are silica and asbestos, lead, arsenic and a number of organic dusts, including those which contain foreign proteins and may produce allergies.

Gases. Some of the most common causes of occupational disease are in this group: for example, carbon monoxide, hydrogen sulfide and nitrogen dioxide.

Vapors. Every liquid gives off a vapor and, of course, many liquids are highly volatile. Some of the more important of those that are involved in industrial poisoning include benzol and carbon tetrachloride.

Fumes. These are small solid particles produced as a result of physical-chemical reactions such as combustion, sublimation and condensation of vapors. Lead and zinc fumes are among the commonest implicated in industrial poisoning.

Mists. These are droplets formed by condensation of

vapors and suspended in the air. An example is chromic acid mist from the electroplating process.

Smoke. This consists of particles produced as the result of incomplete combustion of carbonaceous material.

Smog. This is a combination of smoke and fog.

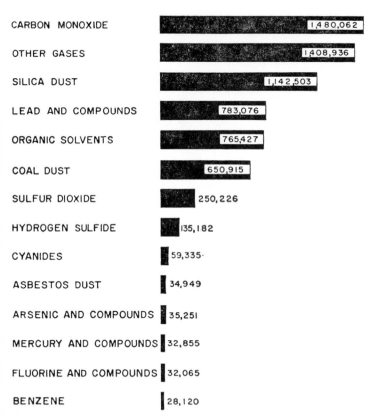

CARBON MONOXIDE	1,480,062
OTHER GASES	1,408,936
SILICA DUST	1,142,503
LEAD AND COMPOUNDS	783,076
ORGANIC SOLVENTS	765,427
COAL DUST	650,915
SULFUR DIOXIDE	250,226
HYDROGEN SULFIDE	135,182
CYANIDES	59,335·
ASBESTOS DUST	34,949
ARSENIC AND COMPOUNDS	35,251
MERCURY AND COMPOUNDS	32,855
FLUORINE AND COMPOUNDS	32,065
BENZENE	28,120

Fig. 29. Health hazards in industry. (Hilleboe and Larimore: *Preventive Medicine,* 2nd Ed., Philadelphia, W. B. Saunders Co.)

Physical Agents

Pressure. In some occupations the worker is employed under conditions in which the pressure is higher or lower than that of the atmosphere. For example, divers work under high pressure, while low pressure is found in mining operations at high altitudes. Pressure changes may produce interference with oxygen supply, disturbance of hearing and, in some cases, air embolism.

Temperature and Humidity. The manufacture of glass and steel requires the use of great heat. Exposure may produce heat exhaustion and heat stroke.

Sound. Boilermaker's deafness is a well-known condition that may affect workers in this industry; however, there are a number of other industrial processes that involve considerable noise which may produce deafness.

Radiation. Exposure to radioisotopes, in addition to naturally occurring radium, occurs in a number of industries. Such exposure appears to be increasing. Harmful results may be due to ingestion or inhalation which may produce marked effects on the blood stream or gonads and, in some cases, may produce cancer. Microwave radiation, ultraviolet or infrared rays may also be hazardous, particularly to the eyes.

Infections

While occupation-related infections are less common in the United States than in the other countries, instances do occur. Examples are anthrax, brucellosis, and leptospirosis, which result from handling skin, hair or animals. Among fungus diseases are actinomycosis and blastomycosis, which may be found among farmers or packinghouse employees.

TYPES OF OCCUPATIONAL DISEASE

Dermatitis

Considerably more than 50% of all occupational diseases are due to substances which produce skin irritation. Greases, oils, solvents, acids and many other materials may produce skin lesions. Protective measures include appropriate skin cover, such as gloves, the use of protective ointments, proper cleansing of the skin after exposure, enclosure of the process which produces skin irritation, substitution of a less noxious material and, if necessary, a change in the employment of individuals found to be particularly sensitive.

Asphyxiation

The most common industrial cause of chemical asphyxiation is carbon monoxide. This is produced as a result of the incomplete combustion of carbon-containing materials, such as coal, gasoline or oil. It has no odor or taste, so that persons are not aware of its presence. It produces its effects by combining with the hemoglobin in the blood, thus interfering with the oxygen supply to the body. It produces headache, nausea and vomiting, weakness, and eventually death.

The other important chemical asphyxiants are cyanides, particularly hydrogen cyanide, although they are much less important than carbon monoxide. Among the commonly practiced protective measures are adequate ventilation, gas masks and respirators, careful control of the industrial process to reduce carbon monoxide hazard, and employee education.

Pneumoconiosis

This includes two important diseases—silicosis and asbestosis. Both are due to dusts. Silicosis, recognized

for many years, is a fibrotic disease of the lungs resulting from prolonged exposure to the dust of silica. It
therefore occurs frequently in mining operations, where
silica dust is common. The subsequent fibrosis of the
lungs eventually produces shortness of breath, the degree depending upon the extent of fibrosis. Emphysema
and cardiac involvement may also result. Silicosis also
appears to lower resistance to tuberculosis, and the
latter disease often occurs in association with silicosis.
The symptoms of asbestosis are similar, although tuberculosis does not appear to be especially common in patients with this disease.

Control of these important dust diseases involves
adequate ventilation, wetting of dusts, and various
other methods commonly used for the removal of dusts
from the atmosphere. Respirators may also be useful.

Lead Poisoning

Exposure to lead occurs in a number of industries including the manufacture and use of paints and the production of storage batteries. Lead is usually absorbed
through the lungs in the form of dusts or fumes and is
stored chiefly in the bones. Excretion from the body is
slow, so that while acute cases of lead poisoning do
occur, the disease is more likely to be due to long-
continued exposure. Symptoms may be referable to the
alimentary tract (including abdominal pain and consti-
pation), or they may be neuromuscular (in which weakness or paralysis may occur, particularly in the arm) or
referable to central nervous system involvement. Lead
may be found in the blood or urine. The most important control measures required for the prevention of
lead poisoning involve reduction of exposure by measures such as enclosing the harmful material so that it

cannot escape into the atmosphere, improved general and local exhaust ventilation, employee education and careful surveillance of employees.

Cancer

Cancer may be produced by industrial exposure, for example, in occupations that involve exposure to radium or x ray. Most occupational cancers are skin lesions which result from long-continued exposure to carcinogenic agents. Beta naphthylamine is an important occupational hazard which may produce cancer of the bladder. It is commonly used in the dye industry; however, its manufacture has been stopped in many states.

There are, of course, no certain ways of avoiding cancer, because it is often difficult for the worker to even know that he has been exposed to carcinogenic agents. Obviously, when such agents are known to exist, reasonable control measures may be taken by substituting another product or by exercising care in worker exposure. On the other hand, it should be a responsibility of management to ensure, to the extent possible, that known carcinogenic agents are not used.

In recent years increasing numbers of chemicals are being used in industrial processes. Animal studies have revealed some of these chemicals to be carcinogenic and the Department of Labor has taken action to require protective measures. It is likely that many more of these chemicals than are currently recognized fall into this same category.

There are, of course, large numbers of materials used in industry which may cause illness. No attempt is being made to deal with the subject exhaustively in this text.

OCCUPATIONAL ACCIDENTS

Industrial accidents are a major factor involved in absence from work. While covered in another chapter, it would not be appropriate to discuss occupational health without some mention of the subject of accidents here. More accidental deaths occur in agriculture than in any other major industry. Almost a quarter of all industrial accidental deaths involve agricultural employ-

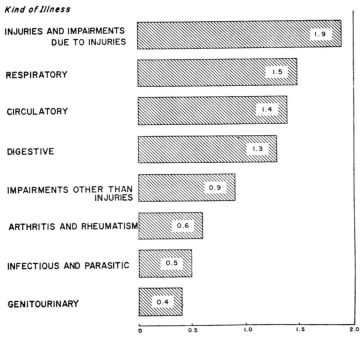

Fig. 30.   Average days lost from work because of illness. (Hilleboe and Larimore: *Preventive Medicine,* 2nd Ed., Philadelphia, W. B. Saunders Co.)

ees. The mining and construction industries are also important in this regard. According to the Department of Labor, there were 4760 deaths due to private industry accidents in 1977. In that same year, Bureau of Labor Statistics data indicates that there were more than 2 million instances of industrial accidents resulting in loss of work. However, it should be noted that the safety movement in industry has been remarkably successful. Noteworthy examples are found in the railroad industry and in iron and steel plants. Control measures involve improved machinery with due emphasis on the reduction of employee hazards, proper training of employees in the use of equipment and machinery and appropriate use of safety equipment.

OCCUPATIONAL HEALTH PROGRAMS

Occupational health programs have as their major objective the reduction of death, disease and disability by control measures aimed at the employee and control measures aimed at the environment.

The Employee Health Program

Pre-employment Examination. The main purpose of this examination is the determination of any handicapping conditions, physical or emotional, which may render the potential employee unfit for certain kinds of employment. The examination also establishes a base line of the employee's health status and may reveal previously unknown defects which need correction.

Periodic Examinations. These are particularly important for workers exposed to toxic substances or other industrial hazards. For example, the worker exposed to lead should receive a routine examination at intervals to detect early signs of lead poisoning; if evidence of poisoning is found, both he and management may be able to take appropriate control measures. In addition, however, a useful service maintained by a number of industries involves counselling of the employee who feels that he has a problem with which the medical service may be of assistance. A good example would be the case of an alcoholic. Many industries have learned the value of early attention to an alcoholic employee for whom that industry may have spent considerable time and money in training. Furthermore, a worker no longer useful, for either physical or emotional reasons, in one type of job may be found to be suitable for employment in another capacity.

First Aid and Emergency Clinic Service. It is clear that in an industry of any size this service is essential. It affords a location where the employee may be seen for emergency on-the-spot assistance for accidental injuries or illness. Management has found that it is considerably more economical to maintain such a service rather than to refer the employee elsewhere, which often involves unnecessary expenditure of employee-time. On the other hand, this service is not, of course, meant to be comprehensive. It involves only emergency care, followed by referral, as necessary, to the family physician.

Health Education. Adequate training of the employee for his job, sound knowledge on the part of the worker of the equipment or machinery which he will use, and familiarity with any possible hazards involved in his employment are all essential if accidental injury and occupational disease are to be avoided. The worker has to be trained in the use of protective equipment such as gas masks and respirators or equipment designed for the protection of his skin and eyes. He must also be trained to exercise personal cleanliness. Clearly, workers using chemicals which may produce occupational diseases of the skin must wash their hand, take showers and have frequent changes of clothing.

Control of the Environment

Some of the control measures that are desirable in order to prevent occupation-related disease have been briefly mentioned earlier in this chapter. It may be convenient, however, to classify here some of the main steps that need to be taken in order to provide reasonable control of the environment:

Good Housekeeping. This is one of the most important steps required on a continuing basis for preventing contamination of the working environment. It is easy in industry for toxic waste materials to settle in many locations in the building. The use of vacuum sweepers, wetting agents and other methods of early collection and disposal of waste materials is essential.

Proper Design of Plant and Equipment. It is obviously easier and cheaper to plan safety features before the plant is built or machinery and equipment installed. Careful attention to construction details and to design and placement of machinery can play an important role in reducing what may otherwise be serious hazards to the worker. It is also essential to maintain buildings, machinery and equipment in good repair at all times.

Periodic Surveys. This is an important practical method of checking routinely on the state of the plant, machinery and equipment. Routine analysis of the air is essential in industries where dusts are common. Other appropriate surveys, depending upon the type of industry or process involved, are similarly important.

Substitution of Materials. One of the ways used to reduce or eliminate exposure to hazardous material is to substitute a less toxic material for a more harmful one. While this is not always feasible, possible substitutions should always be kept in mind, for example, methyl chloroform for carbon tetrachloride, or metal silicates in place of sand (free silica) in sandblasting.

Ventilation. Adequate air changes in the working environment may often play a key role in reducing the level of contamination of the atmosphere. This is particularly true in the case of gases and may be of use to a lesser extent with dusts.

Exhaust Systems. The purpose of an exhaust system is to draw air by means of suction into an exhaust hood. Exhaust systems are extensively used to reduce dusts and gases in the atmosphere. As much of the air contaminant as possible is removed at its point of origin by a local exhaust system. General room or exhaust ventilation can then be used to dilute and remove remaining air contaminant.

Wetting of Dusts. This is an important procedure for reducing the concentration of dusts in the atmosphere. For example, in knife-grinding operations, wetting is applied at the time of grinding. The dust-containing water is then removed before evaporation can take place.

Isolation of Dangerous Operations. Often, when it is not possible to eliminate harmful operations, it may be possible to isolate them to an area where the least number of employees will be exposed. An example is that involving chemical operations which may produce a considerable quantity of dangerous material. If this operation is isolated, only workers directly engaged in the process may be exposed.

Controlling the Process. It should be obvious that proper procedures will often reduce worker-exposure. For example, adequate adjustment of the quantities of fuel and air in engines may serve to reduce the carbon monoxide by-product to a minimum.

Enclosure of the Process. Enclosing an operation so that no air contaminant escapes into the workroom atmosphere is an effective means of eliminating employee-exposure to toxic air contaminants. This method is frequently used in the chemical industry.

REFERENCES

American Industrial Hygiene Association, Ad hoc Committee on Industrial Hygiene, Definition, Scope, Function and Organization, Amer. Indust. Hyg. J., 20:428, 1959.

Baetjer, A. M.: Occupational Diseases and Industrial Health, in *Preventive Medicine and Public Health,* Sartwell, Maxcy and Rosenau (Eds.) 10th Ed., New York, Appleton-Century-Crofts Inc., 1973.

California Department of Health, Bureau of Occupational Health, Occupational Disease in California, Berkeley, California, 1961.

Kleinfeld, M.: Occupational Health, in *Preventive Medicine,* Hilleboe and Larimore, 2nd Ed, Philadelphia, W. B. Saunders Co., 1965.

Traskio, V. M.: Occupational Disease Reporting, U.S. Department of Health, Education and Welfare, Public Health Service Bulletin No. 288, Washington, D.C., 1953.

Chapter 14

Accidents

Accidents rank fourth as a cause of death in the United States, following heart disease, cancer and vascular lesions of the central nervous system. They are the leading cause of death in individuals between the ages of 1 and 35 years. In this connection, it should be pointed out that because accidental deaths occur predominantly in young persons, while deaths from cardiovascular diseases and cancer are most common in older age groups, the total loss of man-years from accidental deaths is probably greater than that from any other single cause of death. Males are involved in 70% of all accidental deaths. It has been further estimated that for every death due to an accident there are approximately 100 serious injuries, although exact information on this subject is difficult to secure. In considering morbidity, it is important to recognize the long-term effects of accidental injuries; it appears clear, for example, that such injuries account for a sizable proportion of epilepsy cases.

Economic loss resulting from accidents is also severe. The National Safety Council estimates that the total cost of accidents in 1976 was almost 53 billion dollars.

Some 50,000 hospital beds are required annually for treatment of patients who have sustained accidental injuries.

Prevention of accidents involves principles that are essentially similar to those used in the prevention of disease. Steps to prevent accidents may be taken at several levels. For example, injury from a falling object may be prevented or its effect reduced by (a) ensuring that the object does not fall, (b) protecting the person against the falling object (for example, by the use of a safety helmet), (c) medical care, including rehabilitation, to reduce the immediate and long-term effects of the injury.

Similarly, injury from nuclear weapons may be prevented by ensuring that such weapons are not produced or, if they are manufactured, by controlling their use. In the event that they are used, the population might conceivably be evacuated from areas which are considered prime attack sites; in lieu of this, shelters might be provided for the people's protection; lastly, steps may be taken to provide medical care to the sick and injured and protection against the hazards of radiation.

Again, as in communicable or chronic diseases, resistance to injury in general may be natural or acquired. The body has a certain resistance at birth by virtue of its structure and form; repeated exposure produces more resistance. Examples of acquired resistance include tanning as a result of exposure to the sun, or the development of callouses by virtue of pressure on the ball of the foot or on the hands. Physiologic tolerance to drugs can be and often is acquired, so that increasing doses may be required to produce a certain effect. On the other hand, it is well known that the ability of the body to marshal its reparative processes effectively tends to decrease with age. In a child who falls and sustains a fracture the broken bones will usually heal rapidly with a minimum of disability. This, however, is not generally true in an aged individual in whom healing is slow and disability common.

The contribution of human behavior to the production of accidents is still a matter of considerable uncertainty. While there appears to be little question that "accident proneness" is a real factor, for example, in the production of a certain percentage of vehicular accidents, it appears that in many accidents there are other factors involved which appear to have little to do with the individual's behavior or with psychologic influences. On the other hand, there is no question but that alcohol is an important etiologic factor in accidents, particularly automobile accidents.

TYPES OF ACCIDENTS

Of approximately 100,000 accidental deaths that occur each year, almost half result from motor vehicle accidents. Beginning in 1962, a sharp increase in deaths from this cause became noticeable. Approximately 30% of accidental deaths, however, are home accidents. Disregarding accidents from motor vehicles, the most common accidental deaths occur as a result of falls, while burns and drowning also produce a substantial portion.

Motor Vehicle Accidents

The death rate per vehicle mile has shown a marked decline through the years. In 1976, there were about 24 times as many motor vehicle accident deaths as occurred in 1910, but there were over 300 times as many vehicles on the road, with corresponding increases in the number of miles driven. In addition to the 50,000 deaths per year due to motor vehicle accidents, about 4 million persons are injured.

Contrary to general belief, motor vehicle death rates tend to be lowest in urban areas. Young drivers have much higher death rates than do those of middle age, while drivers with evidence of certain health defects such as epilepsy, alcoholism or cardiovascular disease appear to be responsible for a disproportionately high number of accidents. Alcoholism is particularly important and is responsible for almost half of all motor vehicle deaths.

Prevention. Studies of speed of travel, increased law enforcement, and the ages at which accidents occur clearly indicate that there is no simple method of accident prevention. Since pedestrians are involved in approximately 30% of all accidental deaths from motor vehicles, it is clear that one of the most important preventive measures that can be taken is to segregate traffic from the pedestrian stream by construction of throughways, turnpikes and similar roads. Accidents involving pedestrians have almost been eliminated on well-engineered roadways. Improved traffic control in congested areas, reduced speed of travel, prevention of "jay-walking," and educating children concerning the hazards of street play are all sound preventive measures.

Medical examinations of applicants for driver's licenses or renewals have often been proposed, and considerable pressure has developed for laws regarding these to be enacted. In general, however, such a program would appear to be rather costly and of limited usefulness. It would be practically impossible to develop uniformity and fairness in its execution, and obviously, in some instances, pressure would be exerted upon physicians to render satisfactory reports. Also there would be occasions in which the physician could not determine with certainty whether or not harm would result from the granting of a license.

The automobile driver's skill, his ability to take proper evasive action and, as has been pointed out, his emotional attitude all play an important role. One of the most important factors, however, is the consumption of alcohol. The reduction of alcohol consumption prior to driving a motor vehicle constitutes an important step in the reduction of accidental deaths from this cause. Driver education, such as is carried out in some high schools, may be a useful preventive technique.

In recent years, increasing attention has been placed on the engineering of automobiles so as to render them more safe. Much more attention will undoubtedly be devoted to this question in the next few years. Safety doorlocks and seat belts are used in almost all vehicles, and there is litle question that they reduce the probability of fatal accidents considerably, since they help to prevent occupants from being thrown from the car.

Home Accidents

Home accidents rank second only to motor vehicle mishaps as the cause of accidental deaths in the United States, accounting for some 30% of all deaths due to accidents. They rank first as a cause of accidental injury; more than 40% of all injuries result from accidents sustained in the home. They most commonly affect persons under the age of 5 and those over 65. Among the most common causes of accidents in the house are falls, fire burns, suffocation due to ingested objects (such as toys), accidental poisoning (including carbon monoxide poisoning) and the use of firearms. Interestingly, the room where accidents are most apt to occur is the bedroom; this is particularly true in the case of falls affecting older persons.

Prevention. Physicians and others should be alert to the various conditions in homes which may be accident hazards. These include the presence of loose throw rugs at the top of a staircase, the exposure of small children to matches and poisonous materials and the use of power lawnmowers by children too young to appreciate their danger. Guns should be stored where they are inaccessible to young children; older children should be allowed to handle them only after they have received detailed instructions and under careful supervision by adults. Improvemnt of housing conditions for elderly persons so as to reduce accident hazards, such as staircases with poor lighting, should decrease the incidence of accidents among this age group.

Poison control centers have been established in many cities in this country and are useful in providing accessibility by telephone to information regarding toxicity of common household compounds, measures to be taken in emergency situations and education in prevention of poisoning.

Work Accidents

The largest category of work accidents occurs among agricultural workers. In 1976 the total cost of all work accidents was estimated at around 18 billion dollars. The most common cause of work injury involves lifting, carrying, or moving materials or machinery; falls are a close second cause. Fatigue appears to be an important factor in the production of accidents. Studies by the Bureau of Labor Statistics have shown that injuries increase disproportionately as daily work hours are extended.

Prevention. Great strides have been made in preventing accidents in industry. Many plants have developed active safety programs in which attention is placed not only on education, but upon the use of safety equipment and the employment of safe procedures. Training programs have also become increasingly important. Proper ventilation in areas where the air is dusty or contaminated with pollutants is essential. Many improvements have been made in agricultural machinery with the establishment of protective devices and other safety features.

Public Accidents

This category includes accidents due to drowning, firearms, excessive heat, lightning, and insect and snake bites. Deaths from drowning are concentrated among children and young adults, and could be prevented if children were taught to swim and to appreciate the importance of water safety practices. Falls from moving vehicles or public buildings or on slippery pavements constitute another important group of public accidents. Defective vision, slow reflexes, and motor disturbances all contribute to the occurrence of this type of accident, particularly among the older age group. Adequate handrails and ramps are useful in prevention. Prompt sanding and salting of sidewalks following snow or sleet would also reduce injuries from falls.

Poisonous snakes in the United States include the pit vipers (rattlesnake, copperhead and cottonmouth water moccasin) and coral snakes. Few areas of the country are entirely free from poisonous snakes. Persons walking through underbrush should be aware of the possibility of snake bite. Heavy, high-top shoes give excellent protection. If a bite occurs, a proximal ligature should be applied immediately, and antivenin should be injected as soon as possible. Allergic reaction to bites of insects such as bees, hornets or wasps are quite common and may lead to severe reactions and even death in those previously susceptible.

EMERGENCY SERVICES

The availability of emergency health services may be a determining factor in influencing the effect of an accident. Since medical personnel usually are not available at the scene of an accident, it is important that members of the public, properly trained in first aid, be able to provide assistance. Unfortunately, too few persons have sufficient knowledge of the principles of first aid. In fact, their fumblings may aggravate the injury.

Since the life of the accident victim may depend on what is done in the few minutes immediately following the accident, organized courses in first aid, such as those given by the Red Cross, should be provided in every community, and intensive educational campaigns should be developed to enlist as many participants as possible.

Every community should have a plan for emergency medical care, which is capable of being immediately mobilized in case of accident or disaster. This plan should include adequate provision of first aid at the accident site, availability of early transportation to the hospital, and immediate expert care at the hospital itself. There must be an organized system for calling the ambulance service and for an appropriate distribution of the sick and injured to the area hospital. Adequate training of the ambulance drivers and rescue squads is essential.

The planning and supervision of ambulance services are a community responsibility, but this responsibility has not been generally accepted. Transportation arrangements for the sick and injured, therefore, often leave much to be desired.

REFERENCES

Accident Facts, 1977 Edition, National Safety Council, Illinois.

Campbell, H. E.: The role of alcohol in fatal traffic accidents and measures needed to solve the problem, Mich. Med. 63:699, 1964.

Larimore, G. W.: Accident Hazards, in *Preventive Medicine*, 2nd Ed., Hilleboe and Larimore, Philadelphia, W. B. Saunders Co., 1965.

McCarroll, J. R., and Haddon, W., Jr.: A controlled study of fatal automobile accidents in New York City, J. Chron. Dis. 15:811, 1962.

National Health Council, National Health Forum (Emergency Care) Summary of Discussion and Reports at 1962 Forum, New York.

National Health Survey, National Center for Health Statistics, U.S. Department of Health, Education and Welfare, Washington, D.C., 1965.

Chapter **15**

Planning for Disaster

While atomic attack may be unthinkable to most of us, it is nevertheless essential for each community to take precautionary measures to reduce to a minimum the disabilities and deaths that would result if such an attack should occur. In preparing a community for such an eventuality, it is important to recognize that the general principles involved can be easily applied to natural disasters such as explosions, serious train or bus wrecks, hurricanes or tornadoes which may occur from time to time. Thus, preparation for mobilization of health resources can be useful in time of peace as well as in war. Furthermore, there is no question that adequate advance preparation and careful planning can do much to reduce the effects of a disaster to a community by its beneficial effect upon morale, as well as in reduction of death and disability if, in fact, disaster should strike.

In planning the steps to be taken in case of disaster, it is essential to relate the medical and supporting health services to other aspects of the defense effort. For example, the availability, type and location of shelters constitute considerations just as important as the arrangements for transportation of the sick and injured. It is also necessary to consider the possible type and size of bomb which might be used in case of enemy attack. This requires an up-to-date knowledge of the weapons currently available, particularly bearing in mind today's rapidly changing and advancing technology. These facts are important because of the necessity to plan for different sizes of disaster areas, which in turn will be dependent upon the amount and type of damage that may be produced.

Take, for example, the possible effects of a 5-megaton blast. From ground zero (the site of detonation), total destruction and death would extend to a radius of almost a mile, with heavy damage occurring to a radius of an additional 2 miles, moderate damage for another 2 miles; light damage would extend to approximately 9 miles from ground zero. Damage, death and disability result from three main factors—blast, heat (and fire) and radioactive fallout. All three of these effects are relatively immediate, but radioactive emanations may extend far beyond the immediate disaster area, the extent and direction being determined by wind patterns; furthermore, they will also last for a considerable time beyond the blast period. It has been estimated, in fact, that dangerous radiation would continue to exist in the blast area for about 2 weeks.

Advanced planning for nuclear or natural disaster requires not only the development of a definite, written plan of procedure, but also, even more important, the proper publication of this plan to those who will be responsible for seeing that it is carried out and adequate training of those who are expected to participate.

As already indicated, the most important immediate considerations arising out of nuclear attack are those of mechanical injury, burns and radiation sickness.

1. *Mechanical injury*

   The effects of blast are most evident, of course, in the immediate vicinity of the bomb and for an area radiating out from this so-called ground zero, depending upon the power of the bomb. For some distance from ground zero, little life may remain, but as one goes further out from this central point, blast effects producing mechanical injury become less and less pronounced.

2. *Burns*

   Much that applies to mechanical injury applies also to burns. Severe burns accompanied by blast would be sufficient in the general area around ground zero to cause immediate death. Small fires may, however, occur at great distances from ground zero so that persons exhibiting first-, second- or even third-degree burns may be found several miles from this point.

3. *Radiation sickness*

   This is an important and lasting effect of a nuclear explosion. The amount and type of sickness and its prognosis will depend upon the dose and length of exposure to radiation. While immediate effects may be severe, long-term results may include genetic effects, shortening of life span and the possible development of leukemia or cancer. Radiation hazards also produce a great need for the development of decontamination procedures. For example, cleansing of exposed skin and the removal of outer garments may effect a reduction in contamination of as much as 90%.

   In addition to these three major effects of nuclear disaster, it is, of course, also necessary for provision to be made for coping with ordinary illness and injury which occur under ordinary conditions. However, in addition, preparation must be made in the event of disasters for epidemics of disease which may arise either immediately or several weeks after the disaster has occurred.

Organization for Disaster

First Aid Stations. These stations will need to be established as close to the disaster scene as is possible, bearing in mind the problems of radiation. At these first aid stations, screening of patients and early medical care, including blood transfusion, are carried out. Since the station is likely to have to deal with large numbers of casualties, personnel might consist of 1 physician, 1 assistant (such as a dentist or veterinarian), 3 nurses, 1 administrative officer, 1 supply officer, 40 medical aides and 8 messengers. The responsibility of the medical aides is not only to assist at the first aid stations, but also to collect litter cases. These medical aides are required to have knowledge of first aid procedures so that they may be able to carry out life-saving techniques, such as the control of bleeding.

Emergency Hospitals. Improvised hospitals may be established in buildings such as schools, provided advance arrangements have been made for the necessary supplies and equipment to be stored in reasonably safe but accessible locations. These hospitals will receive the more serious cases from the first aid stations and will need to furnish, to the extent feasible, reasonable hospital type care.

Public Health Problems. Among the important health problems in planning for disaster are those concerning the provision of an adequate supply of water and food. This is particularly difficult because of the effects of radiation. Water that has been stored, for example, in covered reservoirs or water coming from deep wells is obviously safer than that from streams or open reservoirs. Similarly, in the case of food, that which has been stored in areas not liable to contamination with fallout dust may be eaten. Solid food may be consumed after thorough washing. Nonperishable foods, obviously contaminated, should be stored until radioactive decay has reduced radioactivity sufficiently.

Chemical and Biologic Warfare

Defense against chemical or biologic agents does not seem particularly practical at this time. Chemical defense would require the distribution of gas masks to the total population in advance of attack, while defense against the various nerve gases would appear to be too complex to warrant consideration. Similarly, biologic defense would require advance knowledge of the particular agent being used.

Natural Disasters

Turning to some considerations in planning for natural disasters it has already been stated that the same basic principles apply as in preparing for enemy attack. It is essential to have a written plan of organization and action with a clear delineation of responsibilities. It has been estimated that more than 200 major civilian disasters occur each year in the United States. This type of disaster may be said to take place when the number of casualties outstrips the available facilities and normal abilities of a community to provide care. Advance planning for rescue, resuscitation, transportation and management of the injured is essential if the disaster is to be handled properly.

Many examples could be cited of a disaster which produced utter confusion because the affected community was totally unprepared to cope with it. One such event occurred in 1960 when two planes collided in mid-air over New York City. A disaster call went out to the Kings County Hospital Center in Brooklyn and two physicians and two nurses were dispatched to the scene. The roads were blocked by sightseers so that it took the ambulance 45 minutes to travel a distance normally taking a few minutes. The hospital meanwhile readied itself by clearing wards, assembling oxygen supplies and having available staff congregate in the emergency room. However, when the ambulance finally arrived at the scene it was found that a medical clearing station had already been established in a nearby bowling alley, and the staff was there drinking coffee. It was evident to all that there were no survivors, but communications had obviously broken down and practically no information got to the Kings County Hospital Center.

Just 3 days later, a major fire occurred on an aircraft carrier in the Brooklyn Navy Yard, trapping 250 men below deck. Once again, however, the roads were blocked with onlookers. In addition, unauthorized requests for medical supplies and personnel produced utter confusion. Communications again were inadequate and there was no over-all medical authority designated until too late to be of much value. At one time, 35 injured persons lay on stretchers but received no attention because of inadequate medical personnel and equipment.

A different type of problem occurred in 1957, at Houston, Texas, when a relatively minor radiation accident took place in which poor public information and management resulted in near panic among some of the citizenry. While the exposed individuals apparently received only small radiation doses, attempts were made to suppress the news, thereby producing damaging rumors and sensationalism. As a result, the affected individuals and their families became socially ostracized because of their "radioactivity."

These cases point out that the first essential in planning for disaster is the appointment of one person as a recognized disaster authority and, under his general direction, a single health authority. As a result of this country's civil defense planning a local director of civil defense has been appointed in most communities. Usually, but not always, the local health officer is the chief health authority. Functions of all agencies and individuals must be clearly defined, adequate communications established and a definitive organization with lines of authority spelled out. All health services and activities require program coordinators.

In October, 1962, an overheated boiler exploded in New York City, killing 21 persons and injuring almost 100 more. Ambulances were immediately dispatched and within little more than a half an hour all injured persons had been removed. Early warning permitted a nearby hospital to organize its emergency treatment teams so that 71 persons were admitted and treatment initiated within 90 minutes of the explosion. This incident demonstrates that good advance planning will pay dividends and is the most important single step that should be taken by communities interested in preparing for possible disasters.

REFERENCES

Family Guide to Emergency Health Care, Revised 1963, U.S. Department of Defense, Office of Civil Defense, and Department of Health, Education and Welfare, Public Health Service, Washington, D.C.

Hilleboe, H. E., and Lade, J. H.: Medical Defense against Disaster, in *Preventive Medicine*, Hilleboe and Larimore, 2nd Ed, Philadelphia, W. B. Saunders Co., 1965.

Ingraham, Hollis: Medical Plans for Civil Defense, New York State Department of Health, 'Health News,' 39: 12-19, June, 1962.

Shefton, G. W.: Problems Encountered in National Disasters, presented at Nebraska Health Mobilization Stateline Training Seminar, Omaha, Nebraska, May, 1965.

Chapter **16**

Medical Care

Historical Background

Before the advent of the Industrial Revolution, there were few large cities and the economy was essentially agrarian. Social classes were clearly demarcated and a son usually followed in the father's footsteps. Little industry existed; each family endeavored to produce for itself. The practice of medicine was based largely upon superstition and conjecture. Many medical practitioners were charlatans, and no standards of medical education existed. There were few hospitals and admission to one of these pesthouses usually meant impending death. Most of the medical care provided to the poor emanated from the church.

The Industrial Revolution brought about great changes in the manufacturing process; it also, however, produced radical changes in society. Large numbers of workers left the farms to seek their fortune in the cities. They lived under the most unsanitary conditions in the cities and were exploited in every way. Death rates in the cities rose tremendously. During this era, however, the practice of medicine began to improve. Medical training by apprenticeship was instituted. Medical practice, however, was still in its infancy, while hospitals remained, as before, pesthouses.

Abuse of the laboring classes reached such heights that by the middle of the 19th Century demands for social reform began to set in. These reforms dealt not only with working conditions, but with housing, welfare, education and sanitation. During this period of social reform, the practice of medicine began to make great strides. This was the time of the "bacteriologic era" in which rapid development began to take place in laboratory technology, leading to proof of the bacteriologic cause of many diseases. Medical schools were established and provided formal training for those who wished to practice medicine. At the same time, medical specialists came upon the scene. New hospitals were built and began to assume their place as centers for the restoration of health rather than being institutions to which one was consigned to die. Group practice began, and medical care was offered on a competitive fee-for-service basis.

The early 20th century saw the practice of medicine really begin to come into its own. New scientific knowledge was developing rapidly, and the physician took a course of training in order to acquire this knowledge and utilize it in his practice. Increasingly high standards were developed and the public began to demand more from the medical practitioner. It was also during this period that many of the paramedical professions began to develop.

Cost of Medical Care

During the early days of medical practice, costs of providing such elementary medical services as were then available were relatively small, although still beyond the means of a high percentage of the working

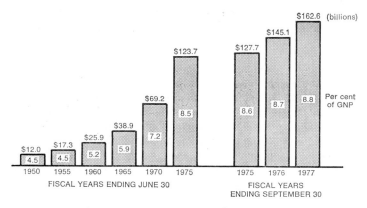

Source: Health Care Financing Administration

Fig. 31. National health expenditures as a per cent of GNP, selected fiscal years, 1950-77.

classes. As medical technology has advanced and modern therapeutic methods, facilities, equipment and drugs have been developed, costs of providing the best in medical care have continued to rise. At this time, it has been estimated that, on any given day, approximately 2% of the working population of the United States is disabled by illness. At least 20% of the population is sufficiently sick each year to require the services of a physician. As a matter of fact, a recent survey of family usage of health services throughout the nation indicated that more than 75% of the civilian non-institutionalized population of the United States saw a physician in 1977, with an average of almost 5 visits per person. In order to avail themselves of health services, the average person spends approximately 9% of his earnings on health care.

On the other hand, it is important to realize that these average figures have little meaning for the individual family. Considerable variation exists in medical care expenditures. Furthermore, similar variation occurs in the ability of families to pay for medical care. While it is true that the United States enjoys the highest standard of living of any country, many families still are able to afford only the barest essentials while others are totally dependent upon government for support. It is also important to recognize that, in general, as one goes down the socioeconomic ladder, the prevalence of human disease rises. Thus, illness tends to strike more often in families least able to afford medical care. This is perhaps even truer as one looks at age distribution. As people get older, the incidence of chronic disease rises steeply; yet, it is the chronic diseases that are particularly costly. Moreover, the annual income of persons above the age of 65 is considerably lower than it it for younger segments of society. This inequity of purchasing power distribution may be pinpointed by the estimate that about 10% of families in the United States pay 40% of the total cost of illness.

It was previously stated that the average person's annual expenditure for medical care now amounts to about 9% of his income. The percentage has risen steeply in the past few years. Some 30 years ago, the figure was 4%. Since then income has greatly increased. While the cost of food, housing and other items have also increased greatly in recent years, the increase in cost of medical care is relatively greater than the increase for these other expenditures. Much of this relative increase has gone into the costs of hospitalization and drugs. As a matter of fact, the proportion of the medical care dollar going to physicians and dentists has substantially decreased over these same 30 years.

National Health Expenditures and Per Cent Distribution, According to Type of Expenditure: United States, Selected Fiscal Years 1950-77

(Data are compiled by the Health Care Financing Administration)

Type of expenditure	1950	1955	1960	Year 1965	1970	1975[1]	1977[1,2]
				Amount in billions			
Total	$12.0	$17.3	$25.9	$38.9	$69.2	$127.7	$162.6
Health services and supplies	11.2	16.4	24.2	35.7	64.1	119.8	153.9
Hospital care	3.7	5.7	8.5	13.2	25.9	50.0	65.6
Physician services	2.7	3.6	5.6	8.4	13.5	24.6	32.2
Dentist services	0.9	1.5	1.9	2.7	4.5	8.0	10.0
Nursing home care	0.2	0.3	0.5	1.3	3.8	9.6	12.6
Other professional services ..	0.4	0.5	0.9	1.0	1.4	2.5	3.2
Drugs and drug sundries ...	1.6	2.3	3.6	4.6	7.1	10.6	12.5
Eyeglasses and appliances ..	0.5	0.6	0.8	1.1	1.8	1.8	2.1
Expenses for prepayment ...	0.4	0.6	1.0	1.5	2.5	6.0	7.6
Public health activities	0.4	0.4	0.4	0.7	1.4	3.1	3.7
Other health services	0.4	0.9	1.0	1.2	2.2	3.6	4.3
Research and construction	0.8	0.9	1.7	3.2	5.1	7.9	8.7
Research	0.1	0.2	0.6	1.4	1.8	3.1	3.7
Construction	0.7	0.7	1.1	1.8	3.3	4.8	5.0
				Per cent distribution			
Total	100.0	100.0	100.0	100.0	100.0	100.0	100.0
Health services and supplies	93.3	94.8	93.4	91.8	92.6	93.8	94.6
Hospital care	30.8	32.9	32.8	33.9	37.4	39.1	40.3
Physician services	22.5	20.8	21.6	21.6	19.5	19.3	19.8
Dentist services	7.5	8.7	7.3	6.9	6.5	6.3	6.2
Nursing home care	1.7	1.7	1.9	3.4	5.5	7.5	7.7
Other professional services ..	3.4	2.9	3.5	2.6	2.0	2.0	2.0
Drugs and drug sundries	13.3	13.3	13.9	11.8	10.3	8.3	7.7
Eyeglasses and appliances ..	4.2	3.5	3.1	2.8	2.6	1.4	1.3
Expenses for prepayment ...	3.3	3.5	3.9	3.9	3.6	4.7	4.7
Public health activities	3.3	2.3	1.5	1.8	2.0	2.4	2.3
Other health services	3.3	5.2	3.9	3.1	3.2	2.8	2.6
Research and construction	6.7	5.2	6.6	8.2	7.4	6.2	5.4
Research	0.9	1.2	2.3	3.6	2.6	2.4	2.3
Construction	5.8	4.0	4.3	4.6	4.8	3.8	3.1

[1]Data for fiscal year ending September 30; all other data for fiscal year ending June 30.
[2]Preliminary estimate.

Sources: Gibson, R. M., and Fisher, C. R.: National health expenditures, fiscal year 1977. *Social Security Bulletin* 41(7):3–20, July 1978; Office of Policy, Planning, and Research, Health Care Financing Administration: Selected data.

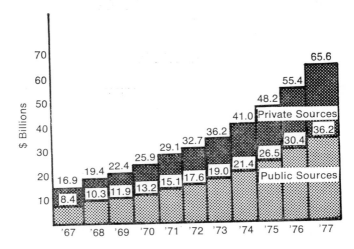

* Total Expenditures are all payments to community hospitals
  and to federal government hospitals.

Source: SSA Bulletin April 1977, Gibson & Mueller, Table 7; July
1978, Gibson & Fisher, Table 3.

Fig. 32. Total expenditures for hospital care:* public
and private sources 1967-1977.

The cost of hospitalization has sky-rocketed. The average patient at Massachusetts General Hospital pays
per hour today more than what the average patient
paid per day in the early 1920's. As recently as 1940, a
private patient paid approximately $10.25 per day. By
1970, this had risen to approximately $100.00. This in-
crease in the cost of hospital care has occurred much
more rapidly than have other goods and services in the
economy. Medical care has been the fastest rising item
in the consumer price index in recent years, with hospital costs accounting for the largest proportion of this

increase; physicians' fees have been second on this list. Public indignation at these costs would undoubtedly be much greater were it not for third party payment. The fact is, however, that most people discover that this third party payment rarely covers all of the cost and, in some cases, will only cover as little as a quarter of the total bill.

It should be noted that the American medical system, in its full spectrum, from the private specialist's office to the municipal hospital wards, has never been able to structure the kind of competitive situation which encourages and rewards economies.

Personal expenditures for medical care have risen from $7.5 billion in 1948 to $50 billion in 1968, $75 billion in 1971, and an estimated $220 billion by 1980. The United States spends 8.8% of its gross national product on medical care—a higher percentage than any other country in the world. Yet, on most objective standards such as infant mortality or life expectancy it is far from being the leader.

In 1950, medical care expenditures represented 4.6% of the gross national product. Higher prices (inflation) have caused almost one-half of the increase. Hospital charges grew approximately twice as fast as did professional fees during the period 1966 to 1971. In 1978, hospitals accounted for 40 cents of the health care dollar with physician costs taking 19 cents.

For the past 25 years or so, financing programs for medical care, whether private or public, have served largely to provide financial under-pinning for conventional ways of providing services. Most of the money has followed well-worn and sometimes rutted roads into institutional cash drawers and medical pocketbooks. Instead of encouraging change, the programs have rewarded traditional methods and old inefficiencies. Nor

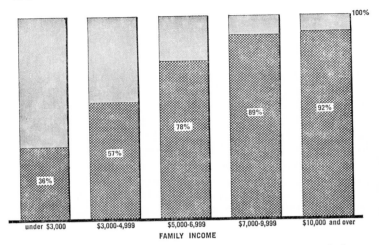

Fig. 33. Proportion of persons under age 65 with hospital insurance in relation to family income. (From Towards a Comprehensive Health Policy for the 1970's, HEW, May, 1971.)

is financing the only problem. As a result of a revolution of rising expectations, consumers are acquiring more informed and expensive tastes. Changes in the delivery of health care services are clearly overdue.

Insurance against Medical Costs

It is clear that the provision of good medical care requires ability on the part of the recipient patient to pay for this care. It has already been pointed out that this ability varies greatly in different segments of society.

Commercial Insurance. Commercial medical insurance plans were first offered in this country at about the middle of the 19th century but did not really begin to grow until near the end of the century. Growth of

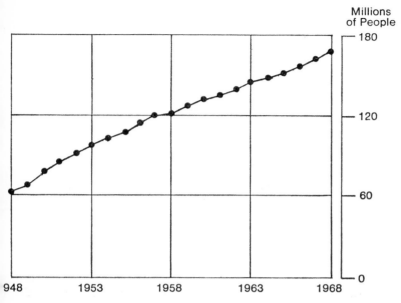

Fig. 34. Number of people with hospital expense insurance coverage in the United States. (From 1969 Source Book of Health Insurance Data.)

commercial insurance has become particularly rapid, however, since the 1930's with increasing attention being given in recent years to protection against costs resulting from prolonged and expensive illnesses. This latter insurance has only become available since the early 1950's. Medical care insurance is provided either on an individual or group basis and benefits available vary considerably with the insurance company and with the patient's age. Most plans are designed to cover hospital costs, but usually even this coverage is limited.

The Blue Cross and Blue Shield plans are particularly

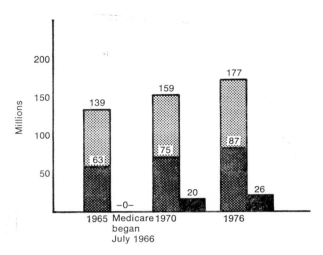

Source: Health Insurance Institute. Source Book of Health Insurance Data, 1977–78 and Health Care Financing Administration.

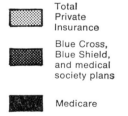

Total
Private
Insurance

Blue Cross,
Blue Shield,
and medical
society plans

Medicare

Fig. 35. Number of persons with Medicare and private health insurance coverage, 1965-76.

Health care coverage status, according to type of coverage: United States, 1976

(Data are based on household interviews of a sample of the civilian noninstitutionalized population)

Type of coverage	Health care coverage status			
	Number of persons in thousands	Cumulative number of persons in thousands	Per cent of population	Cumulative per cent of population
Private hospital insurance[1]	159,957	159,957	75.9	75.9
Medicare coverage only[2]	7,756	167,713	3.7	79.6
Medicaid coverage only[3]	12,162	179,875	5.8	85.4
Other programs only[4]	5,084	184,959	2.4	87.8
Private hospital insurance, but kind of coverage unknown ..	1,624	186,583	0.8	88.6
Unknown if covered	861	187,444	0.4	89.0
No coverage	23,200	210,644	11.0	100.0

[1] Includes all persons with private hospital insurance coverage whether or not they have other coverage (e.g. Medicare) as well.

[2] Includes persons over 65 years of age who have Medicare with no private coverage and persons under 65 years of age who have Medicare with no other public or private coverage.

[3] Includes persons who did not have private insurance or Medicare, and reported either (a) receipt of Medicaid services in the previous year, or (b) eligibility for Medicaid as a reason for not having other coverage, or (c) receipt of benefit payments under Aid to Families with Dependent Children or Supplemental Security Income in the past year.

[4] Includes military (Civilian Health and Medical Program of the Uniformed Services), Veterans Administration, private surgical coverage only, and professional courtesy as reasons for holding no other type of public or private coverage.

NOTE: In order to avoid multiple counting of individuals, these estimates were derived by assigning each individual to one coverage category only. Persons with both private insurance and Medicare, for example, were placed in the private insurance category. As a result, Medicare and Medicaid estimates do not correspond to counts available from those programs.

Source: Division of Health Interview Statistics, National Center for Health Statistics: Unpublished data from the Health Interview Survey.

popular. These are essentially non-profit medical care prepayment insurance plans provided on an individual or, more commonly, on a group basis, to cover hospital costs (Blue Cross) and physician's services in hospitals (Blue Shield). It should be noted that they do not usually cover physician's office services or home calls, nor

Private health insurance coverage status, according to type of plan and selected characteristics: United States, 1975

(Data are based on household interviews of a sample of the civilian noninstitutionalized population)

| Selected characteristic | All persons | Covered—type of plan | | Fee for service | Not covered | Unknown |
		All types of coverage	Prepaid group practice			
		Number of persons in thousands				
Total	209,065	158,085	6,532	151,552	47,433	3,547
Age						
Under 17 years	61,945	45,090	2,010	43,079	15,647	1,208
17–44 years	82,738	64,224	2,664	61,561	17,155	1,358
45–64 years	43,094	35,481	1,451	34,031	6,989	623
65 years and over	21,287	13,290	408	12,882	7,641	357
64 years and under . . .	187,777	144,795	6,124	138,671	39,792	3,190
Sex						
Male	100,865	77,231	3,234	73,997	21,925	1,709
Female	108,199	80,853	3,298	77,555	25,508	1,838
Color						
White	181,874	143,028	5,310	137,718	36,058	2,788
All other	27,191	15,057	1,222	13,834	11,374	759
Place of residence						
SMSA, central city	61,562	43,646	2,930	40,717	16,710	1,205
SMSA, outside central city	82,093	67,464	3,018	64,446	13,305	1,324
Outside SMSA, nonfarm	58,700	42,201	543	41,659	15,604	895
Outside SMSA, farm . . .	6,710	4,773	42	4,731	1,814	124
Geographic region						
Northeast	49,086	38,790	2,148	36,642	9,442	854
North Central	55,892	46,148	763	45,385	9,030	714
South	66,854	46,650	359	46,291	18,880	1,324
West	37,233	26,497	3,263	23,234	10,081	655
Family income[1]						
Less than $3,000	14,676	5,351	171	5,180	9,014	311
$3,000–$4,999	17,074	7,530	241	7,289	9,197	348
$5,000–$9,999	45,273	30,561	962	29,600	14,014	698
$10,000–$14,999	47,103	40,470	1,689	38,780	5,960	674
$15,000–$24,999	48,872	44,290	2,211	42,080	4,015	567
$25,000 or more	20,996	19,395	978	18,417	1,382	219

[1] Includes unknown family income.
Source: Division of Health Interview Statistics, National Center for Health Statistics: Unpublished data from the Health Interview Survey.

do they normally cover dental bills. They also do not usually cover catastrophic illness.

Foremost among the factors influencing the development of voluntary health insurance has been its relationship with industry and labor. Health benefits are now widely available as a "fringe benefit" or wage supplement provided by many employers. For example, the Federal Government pays part of the cost of a health insurance program for federal employees (and their families). Because enrollments are among occupationally related groups, as might be expected, coverage is predominantly extended to those of working age and their families. Thus, the tendency has been for older persons, who most need the coverage, to be left out.

Many of the shortcomings of voluntary insurance do not appear to predominate in some of the comprehensive prepaid group-practice plans that have developed. Benefits are available both in and out of hospital and tend to be quite complete. They usually have the added advantage of being locally administered and, therefore, tend to meet the desires of the membership.

In recent years, as has already been indicated, considerable emphasis has been placed on the writing of major medical insurance plans. These provide a broad range of benefits beyond the usual plans and are specifically designed to provide financial assistance in case of prolonged expensive medical and surgical costs.

In addition to these more traditional insurance plans, a number of specially organized plans have developed which are designed to provide rather comprehensive coverage at home, in the physician's office and in the hospital. These include plans such as the Health Insurance Plan of Greater New York, the Roos-Loos Medical Group in Los Angeles and Group Health Association in Washington, D.C.

It hardly needs to be pointed out that rising costs of hospital and medical care have had their effect on health insurance premiums; these have had to be steadily raised in recent years, again bringing up the question of ability of many of the very people who need the service most to pay them.

While it has been estimated that some 75% of all persons in the United States have some form of medical care insurance, it is clear that coverage varies greatly, and that, commonly, those least able to afford medical care, for example those over 65 years of age, have the least coverage.

Seventy-seven and eight-tenths per cent of U.S. population under 65 had hospital insurance in 1970; 75.2% had surgical insurance. Hospital coverage was related directly to income. For those with family incomes of less than $3000, only 39.3% had insurance, but for those with family income of $15,000 or more, 90.2% had insurance.

Out of hospital services are provided to smaller numbers, varying according to the service. For example, less than half have coverage for physicians' office and home visits, but only about 4% for dental care.

Consumer expenditures for private health insurance in 1976 totalled close to $34 billion and this amount continues to grow.

For persons of all ages Blue Cross and Blue Shield plans have some 36% of total enrollment for hospital care, and insurance companies have 60%.

Major medical expense insurance, geared toward covering costs of catastrophic illness has been growing rapidly. From 108,000 persons protected in 1951, the number grew to approximately 150 million by 1977.

One of the issues currently being widely discussed is that of the relationship between voluntary insurance and the government. Certainly, in the past, the government has concentrated on providing medical care for certain special groups, on providing assistance for the indigent, on construction of facilities and on research and training. On the other hand, voluntary insurance has concentrated on personal health services. Recently, however, this rather clear division has become increasingly cloudy. The most recent evidence of obvious government concern for the segment which has traditionally been provided for by voluntary insurance is afforded by P.L. 89-97, the Medicare Law. This clearly requires the development of a close relationship between government and voluntary insurance companies.

There has been considerable discussion in medical circles, both privately, and also at the government level, concerning the value of group practice programs as opposed to solo practice. The advantages of the former have been cited as producing greater efficiency, better quality of care, increased productivity, improved use of facilities and equipment, a ready availability of a mechanism for prepayment plans, more flexibility in the use of physician's time and in his use of auxiliaries, the availability of in-house consultation and education services, and a more effective built-in mechanism for continuity of patient care.

Group practice has continued to grow in the United States and in recent years, "health maintenance organizations" have been given a considerable amount of both verbal and monetary support by the Federal Government in an effort to stimulate further growth of group practice and prepayment plans. Health maintenance organizations are organized systems of health care providing comprehensive services for enrolled members in return for a fixed prepaid annual fee. Because their revenues are fixed, they would appear to have an

Personal health care expenditures and per cent distribution, according to source of payment: United States, selected fiscal years 1929-77

(Data are compiled by the Health Care Financing Administration)

Fiscal year	All personal health care expenditures[1]	Direct payment	Third-party payment					
			Total	Private health insurance	Philanthropy and industry	Government		
						Total	Federal	State and local
Fiscal year ending June 30:			*Aggregate amount in millions*					
1929	$ 3,165	[2]$2,800	$ 365	— $	83 $	282 $	85 $	197
1935	2,585	[2]2,134	452	—	70	382	89	293
1940	3,414	[2]2,799	615	—	92	523	133	389
1950	10,400	7,107	3,293	$ 879	312	2,102	979	1,124
1955	15,231	8,992	6,239	2,358	412	3,469	1,583	1,886
1960	22,729	12,576	10,153	4,698	525	4,930	2,102	2,828
1965	33,498	17,577	15,921	8,280	683	6,958	2,840	4,118
1970	60,113	24,272	35,841	14,406	890	20,545	13,403	7,142
1971	67,228	26,307	40,921	16,728	964	23,229	15,401	7,827
1972	74,828	28,141	46,687	18,620	1,035	27,032	18,126	8,906
1973	82,490	30,348	52,142	20,955	1,125	30,062	20,178	9,884
1974	91,315	32,989	58,326	23,050	1,220	34,056	22,974	11,082
1975[3]	107,383	33,503	73,880	28,075	2,362	43,443	28,926	14,517
1976[3,4]	122,453	38,450	84,003	32,119	2,625	49,259	33,846	15,413
Fiscal year ending September 30:								
1975	110,665	34,697	75,968	28,514	2,419	45,035	30,290	14,745
1976	126,217	39,425	86,792	33,618	2,698	50,478	34,990	15,488
1977[4,5]	142,586	43,274	99,312	39,299	2,891	57,121	39,823	17,299
Fiscal year ending June 30:			*Per cent distribution*					
1929	100.0	88.5	11.5	—	2.6	8.9	2.7	6.2
1935	100.0	82.6	17.5	—	2.7	14.8	3.4	11.3
1940	100.0	82.0	18.0	—	2.7	15.3	3.9	11.4
1950	100.0	68.3	31.7	8.5	3.0	20.2	9.4	10.8
1955	100.0	59.0	41.0	15.5	2.7	22.8	10.4	12.4
1960	100.0	55.3	44.7	20.7	2.3	21.7	9.2	12.4
1965	100.0	52.5	47.5	24.7	2.0	20.8	8.5	12.3
1970	100.0	40.4	59.7	24.0	1.5	34.2	22.3	11.9
1971	100.0	39.1	60.9	24.9	1.4	34.6	22.9	11.6
1972	100.0	37.6	62.4	24.9	1.4	36.1	24.2	11.9
1973	100.0	36.8	63.2	25.4	1.4	36.4	24.5	12.0
1974	100.0	36.1	63.9	25.2	1.3	37.3	25.2	12.1
1975[3]	100.0	31.2	68.8	26.2	2.2	40.5	27.7	12.8
1976[3,4]	100.0	31.4	68.6	26.2	2.1	40.2	27.6	12.4

Personal health care expenditures and per cent distribution, according to source of payment: United States, selected fiscal years 1929-77—*Continued*

Fiscal year ending September 30:		Per cent distribution						
1975	100.0	31.4	68.6	25.8	2.2	40.7	27.4	13.3
1976	100.0	31.2	68.8	26.6	2.1	40.0	27.7	12.3
1977[4,5]	100.0	30.3	69.7	27.6	2.0	40.1	27.9	12.2

[1] Includes all expenditures for health services and supplies other than (a) expenses for prepayment and administration; (b) government public health activities; and (c) expenditures on fundraising by philanthropies.

[2] Includes any insurance benefits and expenses for prepayment (insurance premiums less insurance benefits).

[3] Revised estimates.

[4] Federal fiscal year.

[5] Preliminary estimates.

Sources: Gibson, R. M., and Fisher, C. R.: National health expenditures, fiscal year 1977. *Social Security Bulletin* 41(7): 3–20, July 1978; Office of Policy, Planning, and Research, Health Care Financing Administration: Selected data.

incentive to keep patients well. In the opinion of many, the development of pre-paid hospital-affiliated group practice programs appears to offer a rational response to the need for high quality medical care.

Government Involvement in Medical Care

Governmental concern with medical care for the poor dates back many years, both in this country and in Europe. Germany, under Bismarck, in the last half of the 19th century, developed a rather comprehensive national insurance program. Since that time, European countries, one after another, have established some form of health insurance program. It is worthwhile noting, however, that since the establishment of a national insurance program in England in 1948, membership in voluntary health insurance plans has grown rapidly, extending to special services and comfort items. It should further be noted that while governments were at first concerned with providing medical care for the poor, in almost every case the government program which was finally developed provided insurance for all segments of society.

In this country, early efforts were made by towns which employed private physicians either at a fixed stipend or on a fee-for-service basis, to provide medical care to the sick poor. For many years, many private physicians have provided free medical care to indigent patients or low cost care to those unable to pay the full bill. On the other hand, public health agencies have provided a variety of services for many years to poor persons, and the extent of these services has continued to increase. Where evacuation of more affluent families to the suburbs has left a higher proportion of indigents in the central part of the city, the city government has been forced to provide local taxes to support medical care for the poor, either at a municipally operated public hospital or by contractual arrangements with non-government hospitals and physicians.

The passage of the Social Security Act in 1935 provided an impetus for more substantial government involvement in medical care. For example, diagnostic, treatment and rehabilitation services have been supported by the Children's Bureau and administered by state and local health departments. While the Federal Government has played an increasingly important role in stimulating the development of health services, many states have developed some kind of medical care program to provide assistance for their needy citizens; an example is afforded by the Maryland Medical Care Program.

In the 19th century, acceptance of responsibility by society in general began to develop. Aged persons who were unable to care for themselves, school dropouts, young men deferred from military service because of physical or mental health problems—all were beginning to be viewed not as individual problems but social ones. Redistribution of society's income was seen as a way to help the poor, and children of poverty-stricken families could be given an opportunity to develop their talents.

During the 20th century, considerable emphasis has been placed on the provision of medical care, first to indigents and to certain special groups of federal beneficiaries, such as veterans, then to medically indigent (those able to buy food, clothing and shelter but not able to pay for medical expenses). The total outlay for health expenditure in the United States in 1978 exceeded 183 billion dollars, of which the government's share was approximately 30%. The passage of the "Medicare" Act, however, demonstrates clearly that the gov-

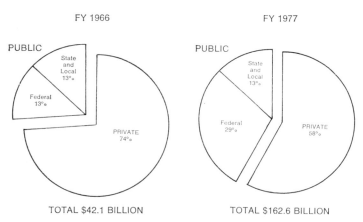

Source: Health Care Financing Administration.

Fig. 36. Distribution of national health expenditures, by source of funds, fiscal years 1966 and 1977.

Who Pays for Health Care

| Fiscal Years | Private Funds | | | | Public Funds | | |
	Total	Direct Payments	Insurance Benefits	Other	Total	Federal	State & Local
			Percentage of National Expenditure				
1929	91.1	**88.5	**	2.6	8.9	2.7	6.2
1940	84.7	**82.0	**	2.7	15.3	3.9	11.4
1950	79.8	68.3	8.5	3.0	20.2	9.4	10.8
1960	78.3	55.3	20.7	2.3	21.7	9.2	12.4
1965	79.2	52.5	24.7	2.0	20.8	8.5	12.3
1970	65.8	40.4	24.0	1.5	34.2	22.3	11.9
1975	60.3	33.6	25.4	1.3	39.7	27.3	12.4
*1976	59.8	32.5	26.0	1.3	40.2	28.0	12.2

*Preliminary estimate.
**Direct payments include any insurance benefits.
Source: Social Security Bulletin, April, 1977.

By Milton Clipper—The Washington Post

Who Pays for Health Care

Fiscal Years	Hospital Care	Physicians' Services	Dentists' Services	Drugs and Drug Sundries	Nursing Home Care	Other Services and Supplies*	Facilities Construction
			Percentage of National Expenditure				
1929	18.1	27.7	13.3	16.7	***	18.1	5.8
1940	25.0	24.4	10.4	16.0	0.7	19.6	3.5
1950	30.7	22.4	7.8	13.7	1.5	16.9	7.0
1960	32.9	21.6	7.5	13.9	1.9	15.7	6.6
1965	33.8	21.6	7.0	11.9	3.3	14.0	8.3
1970	37.4	19.4	6.5	10.3	5.5	13.5	7.4
1975	39.5	18.8	6.4	8.4	7.4	13.4	6.2
**1976	39.8	18.9	6.2	8.0	7.6	13.6	6.0

*Includes other professional services, eyeglasses and appliances, expenses for prepayment and administration, government public health activities, and other health services.
**Preliminary estimate.
***Not available.
Source: Social Security Bulletin, April, 1977.

Fig. 37.

ernment is no longer willing to tie medical care benefits only to those supported by public assistance or producing evidence of medical indigency. The emphasis in this Act is upon providing medical benefits through the Social Security system, thus making persons eligible irrespective of their financial means. While it remains true that physicians, dentists and other professional groups are still primarily responsible for the quality of health services, it is clear that the consumers, and through them the government, are concerned with the financing and organization of health services.

Another change that has occurred during this century is that medicine is practiced more and more in the hospital rather than in the home. Nowadays, the emergency and out-patient departments of community hospitals often serve as the "family doctor."

In spite of the rapid growth of voluntary insurance programs designed to meet the health insurance needs of our citizens, continued charitable contributions, and government support have remained necessary to provide for the medically indigent. Furthermore, in spite of our high standard of living, this medically indigent group now includes a larger segment of our population than just the unemployed or unemployable. In fact, hospital and medical care costs have now reached the point where even a middle-income family, unless adequately protected by insurance, can see their life savings dissipated rapidly by a single costly illness or accident.

The question is often asked, "Does the government have a duty in the area of personal health services as opposed to community-wide programs?" In partial answer to this question, it is not too difficult for us to accept the premise that the public has a right to enjoy health insofar as this is possible. In this connection, it

Estimated health services and supplies expenditures under public programs, according to source of public funds and type of program: United States, fiscal year 1977

(Data are compiled by the Health Care Financing Administration)

Source of public funds and type of program	Total	Health services and supplies										Administration
		Hospital care	Physician services	Dentist services	Other professional services	Drugs and drug sundries	Eyeglasses and appliances	Nursing home care	Public health activities	Other health services		Administration
		Amount in millions										
All public programs	$62,594	$36,199	$7,824	$500	$924	$1,143	$130	$7,184	$3,729	$3,217		$1,743
Health insurance for aged and disabled, Medicare[1,2]	21,591	15,520	4,431	—	457	—	—	362	—	—		821
Temporary disability insurance (medical benefits)[3]	103	74	25	—	2	1	1	—	—	—		—
Workmen's compensation (medical benefits)[3]	2,609	1,315	1,109	—	80	52	52	—	—	—		—
Medicaid	17,103	5,964	1,827	398	325	1,016	—	6,380	—	346		846
Public assistance (vendor medical payments)[2]	517	190	58	13	10	32	—	203	—	11		—
General hospital and medical care	8,296	6,877	21	4	—	3	—	—	—	1,391		—
Defense Department hospital and medical care (including military dependents)[4]	3,392	2,459	91	8	—	12	—	—	—	791		31
Maternal and child health services	637	97	60	15	49	14	19	—	—	378		5
Other public health activities	3,729	—	—	—	—	—	—	—	3,729	—		—
Veterans' hospital and medical care[4]	4,334	3,589	58	63	—	13	31	238	—	302		40
Medical vocational rehabilitation	283	115	142	—	—	—	27	—	—	—		—
Federal programs	42,542	25,715	5,808	310	683	614	66	4,204	1,289	2,424		1,430
Health insurance for aged and disabled, Medicare[1,2]	21,591	15,520	4,431	—	457	—	—	362	—	—		821

Workmen's compensation (medical benefits)[3]	69	45	17	—	4	1	1	—	—	—	—
Medicaid	9,713	3,368	1,032	225	184	573	—	3,603	—	195	533
Public assistance (vendor medical payments)[2]	—	—	—	—	—	—	—	—	—	—	—
General hospital and medical care	1,605	592	21	4	—	3	—	—	—	984	—
Defense Department hospital and medical care (including military dependents)[4]	3,392	2,549	91	8	—	11	12	—	—	791	31
Maternal and child health services	322	50	44	10	38	—	12	—	—	152	5
Other public health activities	1,289	—	—	—	—	—	—	—	1,289	—	—
Veterans' hospital and medical care[4]	4,334	3,589	58	63	—	13	31	238	—	302	40
Medical vocational rehabilitation	227	92	113	—	—	—	22	—	—	—	—
State and local programs	20,051	10,484	2,016	190	241	529	64	2,980	2,440	793	313
Temporary disability insurance (medical benefits)[3]	103	74	25	—	2	1	1	—	—	—	—
Workmen's compensation (medical benefits)[3]	2,540	1,270	1,092	—	76	51	51	2,777	—	150	313
Medicaid	7,389	2,596	795	173	142	442	—	203	—	11	—
Public assistance (vendor medical payments)[2]	517	190	58	13	10	32	—	—	—	406	—
General hospital and medical care	6,691	6,284	—	—	11	3	7	—	—	225	—
Maternal and child health services	315	47	17	4	—	—	—	—	—	—	—
Other public health activities	2,440	—	—	—	—	—	—	—	2,440	—	—
Medical vocational rehabilitation	57	23	28	—	—	—	5	—	—	—	—

[1] Includes premium payments for supplementary medical insurance by or in behalf of enrollees.

[2] Includes duplication in the Medicare and Medicaid amounts where premium payments for Medicare are financed by Medicaid for cash assistance recipients and in some States, for the medically indigent.

[3] Includes medical benefits paid under public law by private insurance carriers and self-insurers.

[4] Payments for services outside the hospital (excluding "other health services") represent only those made under contract medical care programs.

Sources: Gibson, R. M., and Fisher, C. R.: National health expenditures, fiscal year 1977. *Social Security Bulletin* 41(6): 3-20, July 1978; Office of Policy, Planning, and Research, Health Care Financing Administration: Selected data.

should be pointed out that the Federal Government has for many years played a key role in financing research and training so that more can be learned about disease and its treatment and so that there will be a pool of well-qualified health manpower available. These funds were, therefore, provided by the government because it was in the public interest to do so. Furthermore, it seems obvious that a healthy population is in the public interest; thus, anything the government can do to ensure a healthy population is surely contributing to this. Lastly, it would appear clear that the government has a duty to assist its citizens to obtain and enjoy those rights and privileges to which they are entitled, but which they themselves cannot secure without assistance.

Following its role in the fields of public health and protection of the citizenry at large against the ravages of communicable disease and mortality from childbirth and in infancy, the government has concerned itself with other fields of endeavor which have given it a key role in the provision of medical care. Examples include federal support for hospital construction (the Hill-Burton program), funds for research and training of health manpower, the development of a program aimed at locating and treating handicapped children and, more recently, financing of medical care for the medically indigent, culminating with the passage in 1965 of the "Medicare" law and the law providing for the establishment of regional medical complexes to deal with the problems of heart disease, cancer and stroke.

Prior to the New Deal years, Congress and the Supreme Court generally interpreted the Constitution so that the chief responsibility for social welfare was left to the states. However, state governments proved reluctant to undertake costly welfare measures for fear of imposing economic burdens on locally based industries that would place them at a competitive disadvantage in the national market. Thus, the Federal Government, in effect, became the only instrument through which broad social welfare programs could be achieved.

The key legislation which really began the Federal Government's intrusion into social welfare matters was the Social Security Act of 1935 which was the foundation of old age insurance, unemployment insurance, and public assistance. About the same time, the Federal Government completed the first large-scale study of the nation's health, "The National Health Survey." The findings revealed that the poor got sick more often than the rich and stayed sick longer; the poor also received less adequate medical attention.

In 1960, the Kerr-Mills Bill was passed. This created a category of "Medical Indigency" in the Public Assistance Program for elderly people who might not qualify for Welfare, but could not afford to pay medical bills. Then in 1965, the Medicare Act was passed. This amended the Social Security Law to provide a two-part insurance program for persons aged 65 and over covered by Social Security. This provided a basic program of hospital and related benefits to be financed through Social Security taxes. Benefits included 90 days of hospital care, 100 days of nursing home care, 100 home nursing visits, and hospital outpatient services, all subject to some deductibles and co-insurance features. The second part consisted of a voluntary program of supplementary benefits covering 80% (above an annual deductible of $50.00) of physicians' fees, additional home health services, hospital diagnostic and laboratory work, ambulance services, etc. This supplementary program was to be initially financed through a $3.00 a month premium from each beneficiary with a matching amount from the Federal Government out of general revenues.

In addition, the Act called for a greatly expanded Kerr-Mills Program (Medicaid) to be developed by the states but with substantial Federal financial support. This Program was designed to supply health services to indigent persons of any age. Under Medicare, Part A, over 20,000,000 persons 65 and over were covered for hospital charges; under Part B, almost 20,000,000 persons received medical insurance.

Medicaid is a grant-in-aid program in which the Federal and State governments share the costs of medical care for people of all ages with low income. The State sets up a program for this purpose, and makes the necessary arrangements to help people receive the care and services they need. The State also establishes eligibility requirements for participation in the program. Medicaid complements the hospital insurance provisions of Medicare by paying part or all of the deductible and co-insurance amounts for needy and low-income aged people who are insured. It also complements the voluntary medical insurance provisions of Medicare by paying the monthly premiums for beneficiaries eligible for Medicaid.

The Medicaid program, from its inception, has been plagued with rising costs which have been the focus of public (including Congressional) concern. At the same time, a Task Force appointed by the Secretary of HEW reported in 1970 that "the promise of Medicaid that some care would be available to all who needed it has vanished." The Task Force estimated that only about a third of the 30 to 40 million indigent and medically indigent who could potentially be covered were, in fact, able to receive services.

Most persons aged 65 and over have health insurance coverage through Medicare. Complementary coverage for expenses not fully covered by the Federal program is held by approximately one-half of all those who have Medicare coverage.

Medicare patients now account for approximately 40% of all bed-days in general hospitals, a considerable proportion in mental and long-term care institutions, most of the extended care facility population, most of the home health visits and a considerable proportion of physicians' services.

There has been a great rise in federal outlays for health, far outweighing the increases in private expenditures and in state and local government. In fiscal 1965, the federal outlay for health totaled 5.1 billion dollars, whereas by fiscal 1977 it was approximately 47 billion dollars.

In 1977, more than 19 million people received medical care financed from public assistance funds under Federal-State programs at a total cost of some 57 billion dollars. In fiscal 1965, the country's total health cost was 35.7 billion dollars; in fiscal 1978, it reached 183 billion dollars.

In 1977 Medicare and Medicaid combined accounted for approximately 40% of all expenditures in short-term general hospitals. In 1960 private insurers paid 53% of the cost of community hospital care, government paid 19% and private patients paid 28%. In 1976, on the other hand, private insurers and government accounted for 91% of the cost; private patients contributed just 9%.

All of these increased expenditures for health services reflect, in part, improved medical care, enhancement of technologic capabilities and increased access to medical care. They also reflect uncontrollable inflation, overdependence on expensive technologic modalities, and irrational incentives affecting the behavior of physicians and the administration of medical institutions.

REFERENCES

American Medical Association News, February 5, 1973.

Falk, I. S.: The Committee on the Costs of Medical Care— 25 Years of Progress, Amer. J. Publ. Health 48:979, August, 1958.

Hanlon, John J.: *Public Health: Administration and Practice*, 6th Ed., St. Louis, C. V. Mosby, Co., 1974.

Private Health Insurance 1969—A Review by Marjorie Smith Mueller, U.S. Department of HEW, February, 1971.

Progress in Health Services, Health Information Foundation, Vol. XV, No. 3, May-June University of Chicago, 1966.

Putting Health Care Costs Under a Microscope, John Jennrich, Nation's Business, November 1978.

Questions and Answers—Medical Assistance—Medicaid, U.S. Department of HEW, June, 1968.

Rationing Medical Care, David Mechanic, The Center Magazine, September-October 1978.

Report of the Task Force on Medicaid and Related Programs, Dept. of HEW, June, 1970.

Rosen, George: *A History of Public Health*, New York, M.D. Publications, Inc., 1958.

Rosen, George: Provision of Medical Care—History, Sociology, Innovation, Public Health Reports 74:199, 1959.

Social Security Bulletin, Washington, D.C. July 1978.

The Evolution of Medicare—from Idea To Law, by Peter Corning, Social Security Administration, Department of HEW, 1969.

"The High Cost of Care" by Michael Crichton, The Atlantic, 1970.

Towards a Comprehensive Health Policy for the 1970's, U.S. Department of HEW, May, 1971.

Chapter 17

Quality of Care

In recent years, there has developed an increasing awareness and interest on the part of the public and consequently on the part of government in the assurance of the provision of quality of health care services. Just a few years ago, the provision of medical and hospital services was essentially left to physicians, and they were assumed to "know what was best for the patient." Today, however, with the increasing interest and participation of the consumer in health affairs, this traditional role of the physician has been seriously questioned. Obvious deficits in the health care delivery system, concomitant with continually rising costs of care, have combined to produce interest and concern along with mounting criticism of the "system."

As the federal share of the health care dollar has risen, so has the Government's interest and involvement with the question of quality care increased. Surely, according to this view, if the Government is spending vast sums of money to support the provision of health services, it should also develop criteria aimed at insuring that the care provided with these funds is "quality care."

Current concern with the quality of health services in this country can be viewed as part of a continuum of efforts to improve the performance of the health care system. The 1910 Flexner report, which evaluated the quality of undergraduate medical education in the United States and Canada, was highly critical of many of the then existing medical schools, and resulted in the closing of 60 of these schools by 1920. Clearly, however, excellence in education is not synonymous with excellence in performance. Moreover, some 50% of this country's newly licensed physicians are currently foreign medical graduates, mostly coming from less developed countries where post-Flexner standards are not guaranteed.

Present interest in the quality of health services relates, in large part, to the fact that the federal government is now a major third party purchaser of services for the elderly and poor through Medicare and Medicaid. As the size of the federal outlay has risen, cost control has become a major concern of the legislative and administrative branches of government, at the same time that the inadequacies of the benefits of these programs are revealed.

Expenditures for health care in the United States have more than quadrupled since 1965 from almost $39 billion to more than $183 billion in 1978. Concern over increasing federal health care expenditures prompted Congress to amend the Social Security Act in 1972 to provide for the development of Professional Standards Review Organizations (PSROs).

This Act stipulated that the Secretary of the Department of Health, Education, and Welfare should divide the country into appropriate areas to allow for the review of health services provided under the Medicaid, Medicare, and Child Health programs. The Act also authorized the Secretary to enter into agreements with non-profit organizations, preferably composed of practicing physicians, for developing and implementing a systematic review of medical care provided under these programs in hospitals and long-term care facilities. Under this plan, local practicing physicians would organize and operate peer-review mechanisms to determine whether services provided to patients are medically necessary, provided in accordance with recognized and accepted professional standards and provided in the appropriate setting. In 1977, the Act was amended to require PSROs to also review non-institutional ambulatory care.

In short-term stay general hospitals the PSRO is responsible for:

1. Concurrent evaluation, certification, and continued stay reviews to assure medical necessity and quality of care.
2. Medical care evaluation studies to assess the quality or utilization of health services.
3. Profile analyses or retrospective reviews of aggregate patient care data to analyze the patterns of health care services and lengths of stay.

PSROs are required to delegate responsibility for concurrent review and medical care evaluation studies to those hospitals that are willing and able to assume such functions.

Some 203 PSRO areas were actually established covering the country, and as of September 1977, almost 40% of the Nation's 7,000 hospitals were covered by PSRO review activities.

Quality assurance can be viewed as a multi-dimensional process which, as a minimum, requires accurate measures of the technical competence of the provider and mechanisms to improve substandard practices, once uncovered. However, discussions must include consideration of such issues as access to care, continuity of care, the organization of medical services, patient education, compliance, satisfaction, and initial and continuing education of providers.

System-related variables must also be taken into consideration. Such factors as the mode of financing health services, the ease of patient referral and the availability of informal consultation among providers may all significantly affect the quality of services. The financial incentives of the fee-for-service system can lead to over-utilization of services including unnecessary diagnostic and therapeutic procedures. In contrast, prepaid group practices have a financial incentive to discourage utilization and minimize expensive hospitalization and procedures. Such incentives can, however, work against the best interest of the patient and contribute to poor quality of care.

Utilization Review

Mandatory review of the utilization of health services was introduced to hospital-based medical care in the United States as a requirement of the Medicaid and Medicare programs in 1966. This review studies the appropriateness of admission and of the length of stay, and examines the volume of ancillary services used.

Utilization review was primarily intended to curtail unnecessary expenditures of public funds with the hope that it would do so by promoting efficient use of services. In fact, it does generally result in savings, either by determining unnecessary utilization or by denying payment for excessive or fraudulent claims. However, it currently yields little information in regard to quality of care.

QUALITY EVALUATION TECHNIQUES

Measurements of quality of care provided, while highly desirable, have proven extremely difficult, elusive and expensive. There are three overall techniques that have been used; however, all are beset with problems.

Structural Analysis

Measures the quality and quantity of health care resources. Typically, it measures the ratio of providers of health care to patients, accreditation of facilities, types of equipment, etc. However, while this method can determine whether available resources are adequate in quality and quantity to provide the *potential* for good care, it cannot alone determine if the care is in fact of high quality.

Process Analysis

Examines the way available resources are put to use. A typical process analysis makes use of a "protocol" which represents a medical consensus on how a specific medical problem should be handled. This protocol is used to review the care actually provided the patient as it is reflected in the medical record. Because of this, and in view of the fact that patient records are often of poor quality, the process is time-consuming, expensive, and of doubtful accuracy. In addition, there is often no proven connection between process and outcome.

Outcome Analysis

Examines the health status of the patient during or after the treatment process. It reflects the impact of the health care delivery system on the patient himself and is clearly the primary indicator of quality. Unquestionably, if good outcomes could be achieved, it would not matter so much how they were achieved. Experience has shown, however, that studies of outcome have taken years to perform and have been very expensive. A major difficulty with outcome measurement is to determine how the various parts of the health care process such as the performance of the provider, or of the institution, or the compliance of the patient, actually affected outcome.

Medical Audit (Process Analysis)

Most of the research and field work in quality assessment has concentrated on medical audits. This term is used to describe the evaluation of process data from medical records. It is said to have originated with Lembcke in 1956, who audited records of patients on whom major gynecologic surgery was performed, with the object of identifying unnecessary operations.

Nowadays, medical audit is performed by the development of a set of explicit criteria for the medical management of certain diagnoses. These criteria are arrived at either by a consensus of experts or by the adoption of practice norms. Patient records are then reviewed by trained abstractors who note the presence or absence of the items specified in the criteria. Numerical ratings are often assigned and they are then compared to a predetermined standard which has been set for conformance with the criteria.

REFERENCES

1. Greene, Richard: *Assuring Quality in Medical Care*, Cambridge, Mass., Ballinger Pub., 1976.
2. The Staging Methodology: A System for Analyzing the

Quality, Outcome and Cost of Medical Care, Santa Barbara, California, SysteMetrics, Inc., 1976.
3. Report to the Congress of the United States by the Comptroller General, "HEW Progress and Problems in Establishing Professional Standards Review Organizations," Washington, D.C., September, 1978.

Chapter 18

Health Care Delivery

Throughout the past half-century of remarkable medical advances, the delivery system has remained relatively unchanged. Physicians have clung to individualism and old traditions. Hospitals have continued on their own way, striving to be all things to their doctors and patients, creating their own private domains, largely ignoring the need to merge their specialized services and facilities. It is only in recent years that group practice by physicians has been considered respectable and that regional planning boards have appeared to force some semblance of cooperation in hospital construction. In 1967, the National Advisory Commission on Health Manpower reported that "medical care in the U.S. is more a collection of bits and pieces than an integrated system in which need and efforts are closely related."

Although health care is as old as mankind, the concept of organization of health services dates back only some 25 years. Each country has evolved its patterns of health care based on its own history, culture, political philosophy, economy, education, religion, geography, and resources. Evolution rather than revolution has been the keynote by which national systems of health care have emerged. In this country, it has been based on free enterprise and individual freedom of action. A pluralistic system has evolved with increasing government involvement only in recent years. Personal care has traditionally been on a fee-for-service basis with the family doctor preeminent, although this has been changing in recent times.

Center stage in the present health delivery system stands the modern, acute care hospital, staffed with specialists and subspecialists and supported by expensive equipment, admirably suited to diagnosis and treatment of diseased organs and malfunctioning body systems, but nevertheless frequently singularly ineffective in coping with the problems of individuals and improving the health status of populations.

In recent times, few areas of health services can lay claim to have been criticized more than the current ways by which health care is delivered in the United States. Often labeled as a "non-system," the present delivery system has been accused of depriving access to many who need care, establishing hours of operation that make it difficult, if not impossible, for some to receive care and placing emphasis on financial gain as opposed to "what is best for that patient." It has been indicted as a system whose incentives are profit motivated and that discourages cost savings. It has been villified as discriminating against the poor and it has been criticized for providing dissimilar services in rural as opposed to urban or suburban sections of the country.

In most industrialized societies, the general, personal or family physicians are the ones who provide "primary" care, by which is meant fundamental and continuing care. They are the foundation of the health care system. They provide a personal, caring, curing, and counseling service that employs science, technology, essential support systems and other health care personnel as the circumstances require. They are the underpinning of the entire health care system. The primary care physician is in an important position in relation to early diagnosis and assessment. Many of the conditions which come to his attention are minor, transient, and self limiting and may well remain as "symptoms" with no proven or confirmed diagnostic label—cough, backache, headache, dyspepsia, dizziness, and sore throat being examples. However, the primary care physician has to decide what is potentially serious and what is minor; what has to be dealt with urgently and what can wait; what can he manage and what has to be referred to a specialist.

While traditionally, in the United States, the foundation of health care delivery has been the fee-for-service solo medical practitioner, it is no longer likely that exemplary personal health care can be provided by the physician in solo practice. The advances in knowledge that have developed in the past 30 years or so, the resources now available, the diagnostic and therapeutic procedures currently in vogue and the continuing rapid growth in health technology have combined to make it well-nigh impossible for a single physician in private practice to either maintain himself up to date sufficiently in medicine or to acquire and sustain the requisite technical ability to provide the array of services currently demanded by his patients. Even with the growth of group practice, the panoply of specialized knowledge and services available from contemporary community hospitals and medical centers must be readily available to support—but not substitute for the work of the primary physician.

The task of a present day health care organization is

to deploy personnel and resources responsively and responsibly so that patient problems, symptoms, and complaints are recognized at the earliest possible points in their natural history and appropriate action taken in a timely manner. All levels of care, including primary care, consultant care, hospital subspecialty and inpatient care, nursing home care, domiciliary care and their related services, need to be under the control of one organization.

The organization of health services to meet the needs of people also brings with it an obligation on the part of the public to assume certain commitments and responsibilities. They need to accept the desirability of establishing formal relationships with health care organizations or systems. The best known of these is the prepaid health system labeled in federal legislation as a health maintenance organization, under which the patient pays a fixed periodic premium in return for responsible, comprehensive care. In this way, the patient has access to a primary or general physician, supported by a full range of organized health personnel and services. Unless the public is ready and willing to accept the difference between their traditional relationship with a family practitioner and the somewhat more complex relationship that they must develop with a health maintenance organization, and unless they appreciate the difference in the kinds of services that would be made available and the differing costs that may be involved, then this kind of prepaid health organization will not be able to gain general public acceptance and will therefore not really become a viable alternative to the fee-for-service system.

Every health care system has to balance three contending factors; first is the demand for equity or a fair share with respect to the availability and accessibility of health services. Secondly is the concern for the quality of care. Many failures in the maintenance of quality are systems failures not just physician failures. Health care managers must be held accountable for the care provided by their institutions and systems just as is true in the business world. Finally, there is the difficult issue of costs; it is difficult but important to determine whether or not a health care system or institution is being run efficiently and whether the additional costs of providing excess capacity or standby services are justified.

Universities and their medical centers cannot continue to operate in splendid isolation from their communities. They will have to make deliberate and rational decisions on the basis of national, regional or local needs about what kinds and proportions of the several types of health care professionals they are prepared to educate. Medical centers must reconsider the extent of their responsibilities for preparing physicians to care for the chronically ill, the disabled, the destitute and the dying. Clearly, there are limits to the number of specialists and subspecialists who can be suitably employed; they should limit many of their activities to those patients referred to them by primary physicians. They should not provide primary care. Medicine now needs to establish which of its "alleged" cures are both efficacious and cost-effective and see that they are made properly available to all who can benefit.

Among the many responsibilities that devolve upon politicians, the allocation of scarce resources is perhaps the most formidable. With a tradition of piecemeal, categorical approaches to health problems, it is little wonder that resource allocation decisions are often based upon individual sympathy for particular constituents. Similarly, there is need for recognition by federal agencies that health care systems such as those operated by the Veterans Administration, the Department of Defense and the Public Health Service cannot any longer exist in isolation and that there is great need for sharing services, facilities and resources both among themselves and with the community.

Those responsible for making policy decisions concerning the deployment and distribution of health resources must recognize the great difference that exists between the public's needs and its demands and the difficulty that frequently occurs in distinguishing between the two. Clearly, the public has unrealistic expectations of medicine and health care and many of their expectations are unlikely to be fulfilled. It is highly improbable that we will ever have efficacious forms of intervention that can repair all the ravages of time or reverse the impact of a lifetime of deprivation or destructive behavior. A clinically concerned and cost-effective health care system can hopefully help educate its employees on how to use its services in order to anticipate health problems, maximize the benefits of health care and reduce costs.

Health Care Requirements

The basic requirements of an adequate, comprehensive medical care program in a community are:

1. The services must be adequate in quantity. All persons should be provided comprehensive medical care services whenever and wherever needed to detect illness and disability at an early date. Facilities to provide thorough diagnosis and treatment of disease or injury as well as full rehabilitation are necessary. This requires an ample supply of health manpower, facilities, and funds.

2. The service must be reasonably accessible to all patients. There is little value in providing a full array of services if patients are unable to reach them. However, not only is physical and financial accessibility essential, but motivation of the patient to seek care may, in some cases, be even more important. Individuals vary greatly in their personal perception of the importance of health. Motivation is often a key factor in poor persons, whose interests may well be consumed in trying to obtain sufficient food, clothing, and housing to simply eke out an existence.

3. The service must be of high quality. This requires up-to-date knowledge on the part of those responsible for providing medical care. A high degree of professional competence in the various health disciplines and in the application of modern methods and technology is essential. High standards of patient care must be attained in facilities such as hospitals and nursing homes; also required is a well-coordinated progressive care program.

4. The service must provide for continuity of care. There must be a continuum of health services to the patient and his family. The patient must be treated as a whole person, not as a fragmented collection of separate organs. This "fragmentation" constitutes one of the dangers of medical specialization which must be guarded against. Recognition must be given to the patient's emotional and social needs as well as to those that are primarily physical. The responsibility of the private physician in this program is not merely to care for the patient, but to coordinate the full range of health services to be made available to his patient as required. The physician must have knowledge of the available community resources and should refer the patient to specialists, including paramedical personnel, as

required, while always retaining over-all responsibility for the patient's care. The patient should be transferred from the general hospital to the convalescent or nursing home or to home care as needed.

Prepaid Health Organizations

As a result of the conviction that the prepaid rate method of organizing and providing health care services can create incentives for cost savings that do not exist in the fee-for-service system, the Health Maintenance Organization Act was passed in 1973 and provided federal financial support for the development of prepaid health care organizations.

A health maintenance organization is a legal entity which provides specific health services to its members in return for a prepaid fixed payment. They are an alternative to the traditional fee-for-service health delivery system and are designed to provide incentives for emphasizing preventive medicine and controlling the use of health services in order to reduce overall health care costs. The 1973 Act recognized three basic models: staff, group practice, and individual practice associations. The staff model delivers outpatient health care services at centrally located facilities through its own health professional staff which is employed directly by the HMO. The group practice HMO contracts with a medical group, partnership, corporation, or association composed of health professionals who provide health services on a salaried or fixed amount per member basis. The individual practice association HMO contracts with a partnership, corporation, or association which, in turn, contracts with individual health professionals who provide health care on a fee-for-service basis.

Few HMOs operate their own hospital. They usually depend on community hospitals to provide inpatient services. The basis for payment varies from cost-based reimbursement to an arrangement under which the HMO pays each members premiums to Blue Cross which, in turn, pays the member's hospital bills.

The development of these federally supported HMOs during the past few years has been attended by a number of serious problems, primarily financial in nature. The main difficulty has revolved around their attaining financial viability. This has been made particularly difficult as a result of a number of statutory requirements and because of the fact that they have to compete in the open market with already established health care systems. Successful competition has been, to some extent, impeded by federal requirements which have mandated minimum health services which must be made available. Some of these have been quite costly and have tended to place HMOs at somewhat of a competitive disadvantage. However, the number of viable HMOs has steadily increased and this method of health care delivery appears to be gaining in favor and popularity.

OTHER APPROACHES TO HEALTH DELIVERY

Following rapidly on the heels of the social upheaval of the 1960s, the newly established Office of Economic Opportunity became interested in finding ways to bring health services closer to the inner city and the rural poor; the Neighborhood Health Center program was thus launched. These Centers were set up in many municipalities and were intended to serve population groups generally between 10,000 and 30,000 persons, although some serve much larger population centers.

The Centers tended to be oriented to family health care and provide only ambulatory services. It was intended that each Center be linked to a hospital so that more sophisticated care, including inpatient care, may be provided when required. These Centers provide for extensive consumer involvement, even in policy making, as well as in personnel selection, and emphasis is placed upon training local residents for jobs in the Center.

During the 1970s the operation of these Centers was financially supported by the Department of Health, Education, and Welfare which has taken over the responsibilities from the Office of Equal Opportunity. This department has also been involved in establishing centers for migrants and in setting up a number of centers in rural areas under the Rural Health Initiatives program.

In still another approach to health delivery designed to provide medical staff to medically underserved areas, the National Health Service Corps was established. Its primary purpose is to provide financial assistance to medical students in return for which these students owe a service obligation to provide health care in designated medically underserved areas which have tended to have had difficulty in attracting or retaining health personnel, particularly physicians.

REFERENCES

Fry, John: *A New Approach to Medicine*, Baltimore, University Park Press, 1978.

Can Health Maintenance Organizations be Successful? An Analysis of 14 Federally Funded HMOs, Report to the Congress by the Comptroller General of the United States, June 30, 1978.

Health and Health Care "Personal and Public Issues," The
    1974 Michael Davis Lecture, Kerr White, M.D., Grad-
    uate School of Business, University of Chicago, 1974.
Garfield, Sidney: Delivery of medical care. Scientific Amer-
    ica, April, 1970.
Unpublished data from Health Care Facilities Service,
    Health Services and Mental Health Administration,
    U.S. Department of HEW, June 30, 1972.

Chapter 19

Health Manpower

Physicians

Considerable debate has ensued in recent years on whether or not there is a sufficient supply of physicians in this country. Clearly, the number of active physicians has been growing much faster than the population as a whole. This increase is due partly to the formation of new medical schools from 87 in 1963 to 125 in 1980, together with increased enrollment in previously existing medical schools. The number of medical school graduates has risen from 7,300 in 1964 to more than 13,500 in 1976. A further important contributing factor has been the substantial increase in foreign medical school graduates migrating to and practicing in the United States. In 1950 there were some 233,000 physicians in this country or a ratio of 149 per 100,000 population. By 1976 this number had risen to 425,000 or a ratio of 197 per 100,000 population.

In congressional testimony delivered in 1975, the then Secretary of the Department of Health, Education, and Welfare indicated that the physician to population ratio would rise to between 207 and 217 per 100,000 population by 1985. He commented that these

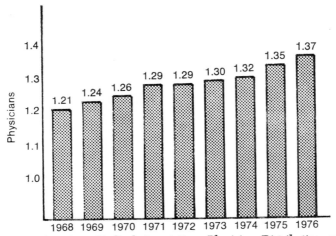

Sources: American Medical Association. *Physician Distribution and Medical Licensure in the U.S.*, 1968-76. U.S. Bureau of the Census. *Historical Statistics, Colonial Times to 1970* and *Current Population Reports*, series P-25.

Fig. 38. Physicians per 1,000 population: 1968-76.

rates would place the United States near the top of all industrialized nations in terms of overall physician supply. These estimates further assumed a 40% reduction in the inflow of foreign medical graduates. In fact, passage of an act by the Congress in 1976 will have the effect of drastically reducing the number of foreign medical graduates practicing in the United States. Similar projections of physician supply were made by the Carnegie Council on Policy Studies in Higher Education in its 1976 report which forecast a physician-population ratio rising to almost 230 per 100,000 by 1990.

In summary, while considerable debate still continues over whether there is a sufficient aggregate supply of physicians in the United States, there is growing conviction that we may be nearing a situation in which we will be producing more physicians than we need.

Specialty Distribution

After World War II, the enormous growth of medical knowledge stimulated by substantial and increasing financial support for biomedical research resulted in a growing movement toward specialization so that by 1975 there were in existence some 69 physician specialties and subspecialties. Concomitant with this increased tendency towards specialization, the percentage of primary care physicians declined from 88% in 1931 to 42% in 1976. This contrasts markedly with the situation in other highly developed nations; for example, in the United Kingdom, approximately 75% of all physicians are engaged in primary care (primary care is considered to include general and family practice, general internal medicine, pediatrics, obstetrics and gynecology).

In June 1973, the House of Delegates of the American Medical Association accepted the premise that there was a need for more physicians to be engaged in primary care and accordingly, adopted a resolution specifying that at least 50% of medical school graduates should enter graduate medical training in primary care in the coming years.

On the other hand, a number of studies have been undertaken to determine if there is an oversupply of some specialists. One study of general surgery stated that the number of physicians entering and completing surgical training each year is greater than required. Studies in orthopedic surgery, neurosurgery, cardiology, and urology also implied that an oversupply of prac-

ticing physicians in these specialties would take place
if the present trend continued.

Some concern exists that an oversupply of some
specialties may produce a number of undesirable consequences. These include the possibility that unnecessary services may be performed and that dilution of the
specialist's skill may occur as a result of his having
fewer opportunities to practice and maintain that skill.

Geographic Distribution

Evidence of concern over physician location patterns
can be found at all levels of government, within medical schools and by physicians, as well as among the general public. It is important not only to have access to a
physician, but also to the type of physician needed at
the moment. Clearly, at the present time, the physician
supply is not distributed equitably in regard to the population. Some areas, such as the Northeast and Pacific
Coast States and urban areas have substantially more
physicians relative to population than do other areas
of the country. This inequitable distribution causes
substantial differences in the availability and accessibility of medical care in different areas. The New England, Mid-Atlantic and Pacific regions rank at least 19%
above the national average in physicians per 100,000
population, while the east south central region is 27%
below the average. Among states, the ratios range from
South Dakota's 78 physicians per 100,000 population to
New York's 198.

As of December 1976, there were 70 physicians per
100,000 population in non-urban areas as compared to
158 in urban areas. This low concentration of physicians
is not limited to rural areas. The disparity is also quite
evident as between inner city and suburban areas. One
study reported that between 1950 and 1970, the City of

Chicago lost 2,000 private practicing physicians—a 35% decrease. During this same period, the Chicago suburbs gained 1,900 physicians—a 130% increase. Throughout the country, the more affluent suburban regions have gained physicians at the expense of poor and black areas of the inner city. As one writer put it, "private physicians are as hard to find in some neighborhoods of New York City as in backward rural counties of the South."

Osteopathic Physicians

It should be recognized that while most people think only of MDs as physicians, there is, in fact, another category of physician in the United States, namely the osteopathic physician. There are currently 14 schools of osteopathic medicine and surgery training these physicians in the United States. In fact, the first osteopathic college at Kirksville, Missouri graduated a class as long ago as 1892. Their standards and length of training are comparable to that of MDs (or allopathic physicians), but they graduate with a DO degree rather than an MD. All states and the District of Columbia recognize DOs as fully trained physicians and surgeons and grant them the same full licensure as graduated MDs. The major difference between the two groups revolves around the importance attached by osteopathic physicians to disease conditions resulting from musculoskeletal abnormalities and concurrent nerve cord pressures and to their belief in the value of spinal manipulations as one modality of treatment.

As of July 1978, there were over 17,000 osteopathic physicians in the United States. More than 50% practice in the east north central and mid-Atlantic regions, Michigan having by far the largest number.

The DOs have tended to emphasize general practice

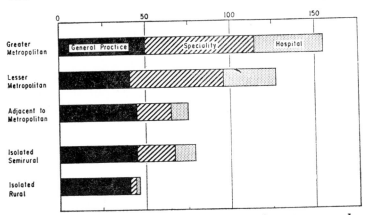

Fig. 39. Urban-rural differences in physician supply. (Hanlon: *Principles of Public Health Administration,* 5th Ed., St. Louis, C. V. Mosby Co.)

and primary care although here, as with MDs, there has been an increasing tendency to specialize. The American Osteopathic Association estimated in 1974 that more than 50% of all DOs located in towns of fewer than 50,000 persons.

Physician Assistants

In recent years, a new health profession has been developed in an attempt to increase physician productivity and help relieve problems in geographic and specialty maldistribution of health care personnel. Assistants to the physician, or physician extenders, can perform many medically-related tasks that do not require the experience, knowledge, and skill of a physician, freeing physicians for more complex procedures and increasing patient loads.

Some universities initiated programs to train physician assistants as early as 1965. Some 900 students graduated between the period 1965 and 1973. However, following the initiation of substantial federal financial support, the number of graduates increased so that some 1,500 persons graduated in 1976. By the end of 1978 some 7,500 persons had entered this field. The length of training has varied according to the institution, from 4 months to 4 years. Student backgrounds have also varied from those with no medical background or experience to registered nurses and ex-military corpsmen with years of training and experience. The most common functions to which they have been assigned following graduation are those of medical history taking and performing physical examinations. Almost half work for physicians in private practice. Some are working in medically underserved areas providing primary care with a physician in an office not too distant serving to provide back-up support by telephone or by personal visits.

Acceptance of physician extenders by the medical profession and by the public has been gradually increasing. Many states now have laws affording them recognition. The National Board of Medical Examiners has developed a national examination which was first administered in 1973. This is designed to certify competence of program graduates. Although they are licensed in 47 states their legal status remains somewhat confused and varies from state to state, making it difficult to know what responsibilities they can legally accept.

Dentists

Future enrollments in dental schools are expected to maintain close to the 1976–77 level, with the number of graduates reaching some 5,400 by 1990. There are currently 59 dental schools.

Health manpower supply and requirements for selected years, 1960–90

Discipline and year	Supply (in thousands)	Ratio per 100,000	Requirements (in thousands)
Physicians[1]:			
1960	259.5	143.6	NA
1970	323.2	157.8	NA
1975	378.6	177.3	NA
1980	444.0	199.3	424.9–427.0
1985	519.0	221.7	481.0–492.0
1990	594.0	242.4	543.0–571.0
Dentists:			
1960	90.1	49.6	NA
1970	102.2	49.8	NA
1975	112.0	52.3	116.7
1980	126.2	56.8	132.5
1985	140.7	60.4	144.7
1990	154.5	63.4	153.7
Optometrists:			
1960	16.1	8.9	NA
1970	18.4	9.0	NA
1975	19.9	9.3	NA
1980	22.0	9.9	22.1
1985	24.4	10.4	24.0
1990	26.7	10.9	25.9
Podiatrists:			
1960	7.0	3.9	NA
1970	7.1	3.5	NA
1975	7.3	3.4	NA
1980	8.7	3.9	9.9
1985	10.5	4.5	12.8
1990	12.5	5.1	16.1

Health manpower supply and requirements for selected years, 1960–90—*Continued*

Discipline and year	Supply (in thousands)	Ratio per 100,000	Requirements (in thousands)
Pharmacists:			
1960	92.7	51.3	NA
1970	109.6	53.5	NA
1975	122.5	57.4	NA
1980	144.3	64.8	144.4
1985	165.2	69.5	166.4
1990	185.4	75.7	190.3
Veterinarians:			
1960	19.5	10.8	NA
1970	25.9	12.6	NA
1975	31.1	14.6	NA
1980	37.5	16.8	41.4
1985	45.6	19.5	46.3
1990	54.9	22.4	51.3
Registered nurses[1]:			
1960	504.0	282.0	NA
1970	722.0	356.0	NA
1975	906.0	427.0	NA
1980	1,152.0	520.0	{1,027.0–1,127.0 {1,155.0–1,326.0
1985	{1,345.0– {1,380.0	579.0– 584.0	1,169.0–1,409.0 1,344.0–1,614.0
1990	{1,484.0– {1,587.0	616.0– 653.0	{1,571.0–1,885.0

[1] Ranges shown represent the results of different models currently being evaluated. Numbers for registered nurses are as of Jan. 1, 1979.

Source: Bureau of Health Manpower in *Health Manpower 94*, 5, 1979.

Note: NA = not available.

The number of active dentists is expected to rise from 112,000 in 1975 to approximately 155,000 by 1990. The national ratio of 52 active dentists per 100,000 population in 1975 is projected to increase to 63 in 1990. This number should be fairly close to established requirements, taking into consideration the role of dental auxiliaries.

The establishment of comprehensive dental benefits under a National Health Insurance program could, however, alter the picture.

Nurses

It was not until 1886, after the value of nursing care in hospitals and in private homes had been demonstrated that community nursing began to develop. It commenced as the provision of nursing care at home to the sick poor. It was soon recognized that an important element in this care lay in teaching family members in the home to take care of patients between nurse visits. This was followed soon thereafter, by instruction in personal hygiene, sanitary measures, and aspects of healthful living for the entire family. Patients tended to be charged a fee according to their ability to pay and the nurses maintained strict professional relationships with physicians.

By 1900 there were some 20 district nursing organizations employing 200 nurses, mostly in large cities. With the introduction of the automobile and the subsequent lessening of the rural dwellers' isolation, the further development of community nursing was enhanced at the same time as the demand for nurses was growing. During this period, schools of nursing proliferated. Public health nursing grew in response to theories relating to the control of communicable diseases by enforcement of isolation and quarantine procedures as well as an increasing role in health promotion and disease prevention activities.

By 1920, all the states and most large cities had health departments in which the largest proportion of professional workers were public health nurses. The importance of health education was becoming recognized and the passage of the Sheppard- Towner Act in 1924 gave impetus to health promotion for mothers and infants. The 1930s saw the development of psychiatric nursing and this became an important function for community nurses. The pattern of nursing education slowly began to change from the 3-year hospital based RN diploma to increasing development of 4-year collegiate baccalaureate programs and subsequently to the establishment of 2-year associate degree programs, primarily resulting from perceived nursing manpower shortages.

The 1935 Social Security Act provided a considerable expansion in the number of public health nurses who were introduced to families who had previously been unaware of their existence. By the late 1940s and early 1950s there was general agreement on the desirability of having one public health nurse to 5,000 persons if bedside nursing care was not being offered; otherwise 1 nurse to every 2,500 persons was appropriate.

In 1964 the American Nurses Association defined a public health nurse as a graduate from a baccalaureate program in nursing accredited by the National League for Nursing, although, it must be conceded that many nurses employed in community nursing do not meet this definition.

With the clamor by people for health services that would meet their needs and the changing role of government in the delivery of health care came the development of physician assistants and nurse practitioners. The latter have received educational preparation either through short-term continuing education, or through masters degree programs. They have played an increasing role in helping provide medical care by relieving physicians to perform tasks for which they are particularly trained. In many rural areas, where physicians were in short supply, the nurse practitioner became the key individual supplying primary health services, usually supported by a physician at a more distant location, who was commonly available for telephone consultation.

In 1976 it was estimated that there were 961,000 employed registered nurses in the United States. According to the Division of Nursing of the U.S. Public Health Service, 1,100,000 registered nurses will be needed by 1980. Data for 1972 indicates that almost 30% of registered nurses are not employed in nursing. Almost two-thirds of all employed registered nurses are employed in hospitals. The most important reasons cited by nurses for not working: small children at home, opposition of husbands, and preference for homemaking. In 1974 there were 58,000 registered nurses working in community health settings including schools.

A few comments should be made concerning the role of the public health nurse today. These nurses utilize their knowledge and skills independently and in collaboration with others for diagnosing individual, group, and community health states. They identify needs for education, preventive and rehabilitative services, and help mobilize community action for development and change. They plan, provide, and supervise health services and they help individuals, families, and communities to develop and utilize their potential for healthful living; they also provide nursing care for the sick and disabled in their homes. In addition to individual patient and family visits, public health nurses work with neighborhood groups having common interests and health needs and they utilize group work skills with preschool children and parents, prenatal patients, and teacher and parent groups. They also work with school age children and adolescents who are in trouble with their families and school personnel. These involvements afford extensive opportunity for public health education directed toward the promotion of mental health.

Optometrists

Optometrists examine the eyes and related structures to determine the presence of any visual, muscular, neurologic, or other abnormalities. They prescribe and adapt lenses or other optical aids and may use visual training aids to preserve or restore maximum efficiency of vision. Most optometrists fit and supply the eyeglasses they prescribe. They do not make definitive diagnosis of or treat eye diseases nor do they perform surgery, unlike ophthalmologists.

The important role that this profession plays in community vision programs should not be overlooked. Optometrists are active participants in vision screening programs among school children and in glaucoma testing programs for adults. They provide visual training and, in many areas of the country, help establish criteria for appraising and techniques for enhancing visual performance both on our highways and in industry. They bring to the health team expertise in functional vision and in the diagnosis and treatment of non-pathologic eye conditions; they also refer many patients to other health specialists when their examination reveals evidence of ocular pathologic condition or systemic disease.

The number of actively employed optometrists in the United States in 1973 was approximately 19,300 of

Changes in the supply of health manpower, selected years, 1960–90

Discipline	1960–75 changes			1975–90 changes		
	Number	Per cent	Ratio	Number	Per cent	Ratio
Physicians	119,000	46	23	215,000	57	37
Dentists	21,900	24	5	42,500	38	2
Optometrists	3,800	24	4	6,800	34	17
Podiatrists	300	4	−13	5,200	71	50
Pharmacists	29,800	32	12	62,900	51	32
Veterinarians	11,600	59	35	23,800	77	53
Registered nurses ..	402,000	80	51	[1]578,000–681,000	64–75	44–53

[1] Ranges shown for requirements represent the results of different models currently being evaluated. Numbers are as of Jan. 1.
Source: Bureau of Health Manpower, Public Health Reports.

whom some 77% were self employed. There are currently 12 accredited colleges of optometry all requiring a 6-year period of instruction leading to a doctor of optometry degree (OD). This includes a minimum of 2 years of college plus 4 years of professional training in a school of optometry.

There are currently some 900 graduates each year and this number is expected to rise moderately for the next few years.

It appears likely that, for the foreseeable future, the supply of optometrists will be approximately in line with the number required.

Pharmacists

This is the health profession that assures safety, efficacy, and efficiency in the processing, storage, prescribing, compounding, dispensing, delivery, administration, and use of drugs and related articles. As of January 1973 there were almost 133,000 practicing pharmacists in the United States. A minimum of 5 years of study is required for a bachelor's degree in pharmacy, including 1 to 2 years of college. There are currently 74 accredited colleges of pharmacy in this country.

The number of pharmacists is expected to rise to some 185,000 by 1990, a number which would produce a ratio of 76 pharmacists per 100,000 population. Indications are that this would be close to the anticipated requirements.

The pharmacist should be used in roles that bring his technical knowledge and skill to bear on some phase of health care. This ranges from consultation with the physician or nurse, to monitoring the course of drug therapy, preparing special forms of medication, such as parenteral admixtures and radioisotopes, and providing an organized drug information service. On the other hand, the use of ancillary support personnel should be encouraged. Many distributive dispensing and clerical functions can be assumed by such personnel, thereby permitting deployment of the pharmacist to the wards, outpatient clinics, and extended care facilities. In addition, pharmacists may be assigned to teams which provide home health services or may help staff community health centers in both urban and rural areas. He should also play a key role in drug utilization, review and control.

Podiatrists

This profession is concerned with the examination, diagnosis, prevention, treatment and care of conditions and functions of the human foot by medical and surgical means. As of 1974 there were more than 7,100 practicing podiatrists in the United States, mostly self employed. They tend to be concentrated in large cities in heavily populated States. There are 6 accredited colleges of podiatric medicine which require a minimum of 2 years of college, followed by 4 years of professional training leading to a DPM degree.

The supply of podiatrists is projected to grow to some 12,500 by 1990. However, it is likely that this number may still fall somewhat short of requirements.

REFERENCES

Report to the Congress by the Comptroller General of the United States, "Progress and Problems in Training and Use of Assistants to Primary Care Physicians," Washington, D.C., April 1975.

Report to the Congress by the Comptroller General of the United States, "Are Enough Physicians of the Right Types Trained in the United States?," Washington, D.C., May 1978.

Report to the Congress by the Comptroller General of the United States, "Progress and Problems in Improving the Availability of Primary Care Providers in Underserved Areas," Washington, D.C. Aug. 1978.

Where All Those Physician Assistants Came From, Marion Kirchner, Medical Economics, Dec. 25, 1978.

Community Health Nursing Evolution and Process, Tinkham and Voorhies, New York, 1977.

Facts About Nursing 76–77, American Nurses Association, Kansas City, Missouri, 1977.

Health Resource Statistics, U.S. Department of Health, Education, and Welfare, Washington, D.C., 1975.

Health Manpower for the Nation—A Look Ahead at the Supply and the Requirements, Howard V. Stambler, Public Health Reports, Hyattsville, Md., Jan.–Feb. 1979.

Institutional Pharmacy Practice in the 1970's. HEW, August, 1972.

Optometry's Responsibility in the Field of Public Health, Rosenbloom, Alfred, Jr., O.D., Optical Journal Review, 1960.

The Role of Vision Care in Society Today and in the Future, Unpublished Paper by Wolfberg, Melvin, D., O.D., July, 1971.

Chapter **20**

Health Planning

While the practicing physician has traditionally been the nucleus around which medical care has tended to revolve and the community hospital has been looked upon as being the main facility for in-patient care of his patients, many changes have occurred during the 20th century which have affected this pattern.

Health resources have not been and still are not equally available to all segments of our population. There are, for example, major geographic variations brought about mostly because physicians, and particularly specialists, tend to concentrate in and around our major metropolitan centers. This, in turn, has contributed to the development of hospitals in these same areas. Furthermore, hospitals have frequently been built with little thought for area-wide planning. In other words, hospitals have often been built too close to each other in some areas, while in others, at the same time, a deficiency of hospital beds exists.

Contemporary planning in the health field in the United States should probably be dated from passage of the Hill-Burton Program which was enacted in 1946. This act authorized grants to states for surveying state needs and developing plans for the construction of hospital and health centers and for assisting in the construction and equipping of these facilities. It represented a major effort by the federal government to increase health resources in underserved areas.

Over the years, the focus of the program has changed from the original objective which was to establish general hospitals in rural areas where previously there were none. Later, emphasis was placed on constructing long-term care facilities for the growing number of chronically ill and aged. In recent years, obsolete urban inpatient facilities have been modernized, while most recently, as a result of the importance being attached to ambulatory care services as an alternative to hospitalization, increasing attention has been placed on the construction of outpatient facilities.

In 1948, 78% of Hill-Burton funds were used for construction of new facilities, whereas in the 1972 fiscal year, 98% of these funds were spent on modernization or replacement of existing facilities.

1965 saw the passage of the Regional Medical Program (RMP) which was to establish regional cooperative agreements among health care facilities, medical schools, and research institutions in order to make available to participants advances in the diagnosis and treatment of heart disease, cancer, stroke, and kidney disease. This program was allowed to expire in 1974.

Not only are hospitals needed for the acutely ill patient, but chronic disease hospitals, nursing home facilities and home health services are also required. Adequate laboratory and rehabilitation facilities, too, are essential.

The hospital emergency room has been confronted by a tremendous and increasing demand for service as the availability of general practitioners at all hours of the day and night has declined. Their physical facilities have become over-taxed—they were not designed to cope with such numbers of patients—and their staffing has been generally inadequate. A specialty of "emergency care physicians" has developed and is growing rapidly as more and more young physicians express an interest in working "where the action is." Hospital outpatient clinics have been exemplified by impersonal attention, long waiting periods often on cold hard benches, and restricted and variable clinic hours—no night clinics and lack of consideration for the patient as a person.

Many of the residents and interns who staff our hospitals are foreign born and foreign trained. While some of them are excellent physicians, the language problem is often a serious barrier to the provision of care.

Evidence that we are making poor use of our health care resources has been accumulating for some time. It has been estimated, for example, that 75% of the pediatric tasks performed by a physician could be done by a properly trained child health assistant. It is clear that ex-medical corpsmen with some additional training can assume a large number of tasks now performed by physicians.

It has been demonstrated that a chair-side assistant, efficiently used, can increase a dentist's productivity by 50%.

It is clear that, in the light of the facts already mentioned in connection with physicians and hospitals, and bearing in mind the inability of large segments of our population to pay for medical care, adequate resources, in terms of both physical facilities and health manpower, are simply not available to all of our population at the present time.

Federal Legislation

Primarily as a result of the belief that unrestrained development of health resources, particularly hospitals and nursing homes, contributes significantly to the problem of unnecessary and excessive health care costs, the Comprehensive Health Planning Act was passed in 1966. The most important purpose of this legislation was to establish a framework for exercising some control over the future development of health care institutions. The act provided for the establishment of health planning agencies covering the country whose purposes were to:

1. Identify health needs and assess available resources for meeting those needs.
2. Establish goals and objectives showing unmet health needs.
3. Assign priorities for meeting health needs through available or new resources.
4. Develop short- and long-term policies and actions for meeting identified health needs through public, voluntary, or private efforts.
5. Develop criteria for evaluating health programs and their contributions toward attaining established health goals and objectives.

In developing a health plan for each area of the country, the planning agency was supposed to take into account the health problems and needs of all geographic, social, cultural, economic, and educational segments of the community.

The health planning agency was also required to review and comment on applications for financial assistance for health-related projects under certain federal programs before the applications were submitted to the responsible federal agency. The purpose of this review was to endeavor to ensure that any proposed project was in conformity with the goals, practices, and needs of the local community as seen through the eyes of the health planning agency.

Undoubtedly, the most controversial function of the health planning agency involved its review and approval responsibility for health facility construction projects. This was exercised through certificate of need legislation which quickly became enacted by most of the states in order to ensure that health facilities were properly distributed and to prevent the development of unneeded facilities and services.

The law also spelled out requirements for membership on the boards of the health planning agencies and specifically mandated substantial consumer representation.

Almost from their inception, the health planning agencies encountered almost insurmountable obstacles to their effective functioning. There was frequent conflict on the agency board between providers and consumers. Previously existing health agencies and professional groups often ignored the very existence of the planning agency. This was often rendered easier by the fact that the meager staff of the health planning agency was no match for the sophistication of those health agencies already in place, primarily funded through local tax funds and having the support of those in local political office. Frequently, the health planning agency was not given the opportunity to comment on proposed health projects; in fact, it was often not aware of projects about to get underway. Often the agency had no effective basis on which to determine needs for specific projects. Finally, many agencies found themselves in a political vise which made it extremely difficult to comment adversely on projects that would bring federal funds to the community and create additional job opportunities.

Health Systems Agencies

In 1975, the Comprehensive Health Planning legislation was replaced by the National Health Planning and Resources Development Act under which the country was subsequently divided into 205 health service areas, each having a so called health systems agency. Many of these agencies were formed by restructuring the health planning agency; others were totally new creations. The act identified a series of national health priorities, as follows:

1. Providing primary care services for medically underserved populations, especially for those which are located in rural or economically depressed areas.
2. Developing multi-institutional systems for coordination of institutional health services.
3. Developing medical group practices, health maintenance organizations, and other organized systems for the provision of health care.
4. Training and increased use of physician assistants, especially nurse clinicians.
5. Developing multi-institutional arrangements for sharing of support services necessary to all health service institutions.
6. Promoting activities to improve the quality of health services.
7. Developing health service institutions with the capacity to provide various levels of care (including intensive care, acute general care, and extended care).

8. Promoting activities to prevent disease, including studies of nutrition and environmental factors affecting health.
9. Adopting uniform cost accounting, simplified reimbursement and improved management procedures for health service institutions.
10. Developing effective methods of educating the general public concerning proper personal health care and methods for effective use of available health services.

Each of the health system agencies developed under the act has a governing board consisting of a majority of consumers rather than providers of health care. Their primary purpose is to improve the health status of residents of their health service area, increase the accessibility, acceptability, continuity, and quality of the health services provided, restrain increases in the cost of providing health services, and prevent unnecessary duplication of health resources. One of their important functions is to review and make recommendations to state agencies regarding the need for new institutional health services, as well as reviewing at least every 5 years all institutional health services in their area and making recommendations to the state agency regarding the appropriateness of those services.

The passage of the National Health Planning and Resources Development Act, like its predecessor, was fraught with controversy and has led to several legal challenges questioning its constitutionality or challenging the health system agency or area designation, or questioning the validity of the governing board designation. Clearly, the potential power and authority of the health system agencies represent a threat to many and portend continuing controversy over the next several years. The goal of restraining health care costs while improving accessibility to health care, while laudable, does not, in the opinion of many, seem capable of achievement. Meanwhile, local health professional groups and public officials continue to question the authority and ability of health system agencies to accomplish their goals.

An example of the difficulties besetting health system agencies is afforded by the number of computerized tomography scanners being acquired throughout the country. These expensive machines, each costing in excess of $500,000 could obviously lead to increased health care costs. Yet, in the absence of definitive standards and criteria, health system agencies have little basis on which to disapprove a hospital's request for the purchase of one of these machines.

A different example involving the difficulties confronting health system agencies in securing closure of hospital beds is afforded by the following New York experience. In the fall of 1977 after a 4-year review of obstetrical beds in the Rochester area, the Finger Lakes Health Systems Agency recommended the elimination of five obstetrical units. Nevertheless, during visits to that region over the next several months, the Governor stated that two of the units would not be closed. Shortly thereafter, the State's Office of Health Systems Management announced that for at least another 18 months none of those beds would be closed because the "personal factor" had not received proper weight in the State's deliberations.

Another problem presented to health system agencies is that they are precluded from exercising any control over Federal health care facilities. Obviously, then, federal facilities operate under different guidelines; yet the expansion of these facilities may have a significant impact on the non-federal system. A recent Institute of Medicine study points out that over 3 million dependents of military personnel are now covered in a program that provides health care in the private sector —the CHAMPUS program. Similarly the construction of a Veterans Administration hospital may have a significant impact on admissions to non-federal hospitals in the area, leading to lowered hospitalization in those facilities and higher per-diem costs.

REFERENCES

1. Report to the Congress "Comprehensive Health Planning as Carried Out by State and Areawide Agencies in Three States," Comptroller General of the United States, Washington, D.C., April 1974.
2. Report to the Congress "Status of the Implementation of the National Health Planning and Resources Development Act of 1974," Comptroller General of the United States, Washington, D.C., November 1978.
3. Report to the Congress "Controlling the Supply of Hospital Beds," Institute of Medicine, National Academy of Sciences, Washington, D.C., October 1976.
4. An Alternative Approach to Hospital Cost Control: The Rochester Project, A. A. Sorensen and E. W. Saward, Public Health Reports, Vol. 93, No. 4, Washington, D.C., July-August 1978.

Chapter 21

Organization of Health Services

While government has long been considered to have an important role to play in the field of health, few persons, even a decade or two ago, would have thought that the role of government would reach the proportions that obtain today. One has only to review the activities of a medical school or school of public health to note the considerable extent to which those centers of learning have become dependent upon the Federal Government for financial support.

It is clear then, that the role of government in the field of health has undergone considerable change. While the earliest attempts concerned themselves particularly with the prevention of communicable diseases within a community, between communities, throughout the country or even between countries, emphasis has tended to change concomitant with the changing health problems and needs of the people.

Governmental health activities have, for the most part, concerned themselves with the development of health services which require organized community action rather than with those services which can be individualized easily. Even here, though, the line between private enterprise and government effort has become an increasingly difficult one to define.

Our modern public health organizations have a great variety of responsibilities, much beyond those concerning the control of communicable diseases. They now concern themselves with such diverse activities as mental health, crippled children's services, health hazards of the environment, medical care of the indigent, home health services, and even problems of chronic diseases, particularly in older citizens.

To cope with these ever increasing responsibilities, the organization of governmental health services has changed greatly over the years. Before discussing this organization in the United States, however, it is appropriate to discuss the organization of health services on an international level. This is particularly germane in light of the considerable contribution of this country in supporting the international effort, with both funds and personnel.

HEALTH SERVICES AT THE INTERNATIONAL LEVEL

World Health Organization

This is the major international health agency. Its headquarters' office is located in Geneva, Switzerland; it also has several regional offices, that for the Western Hemisphere being located in Washington, D.C., and known as the Pan-American Health Organization. The functions of the World Health Organization are chiefly:

1. To help countries throughout the world to improve their own health services. This may be accomplished in a variety of ways; for example, the World Health Organization may, upon request, send a team of public health specialists to help control malaria in a particular country or even on a whole continent.

2. To endeavor to coordinate health programs throughout the world by seeking the assistance of nations in helping each other raise health standards.
3. To provide a variety of specialized services to member nations, including epidemiologic reporting, statistical data concerning the prevalence of particular diseases, standardization of public health procedures and drugs, and health informational materials.
4. To operate an extensive program of education and training in the health field. For example, a country may request the World Health Organization to assign a public health specialist to that country to serve as an instructor at a university.
5. To carry on a variety of research programs aimed at acquiring new or improved information concerning communicable diseases, nutrition, methods of health administration, etc.

The World Health Organization has placed great stress on programs such as malaria, tuberculosis and venereal disease control, maternal and child health, nutrition and environmental health.

HEALTH SERVICES AT THE FEDERAL LEVEL

The organization of the Federal Government in the field of health has undergone many changes during the past few years. In part, these changes have resulted from the remarkable increase in governmental involvement, particularly in medical care and the delivery of health services.

For many years, the dominant Federal health agency in the United States was the United States Public Health Service, a semi-military organization which was essentially operated by a Commissioned Officer Corps. Actions taken during the past few years, however, have

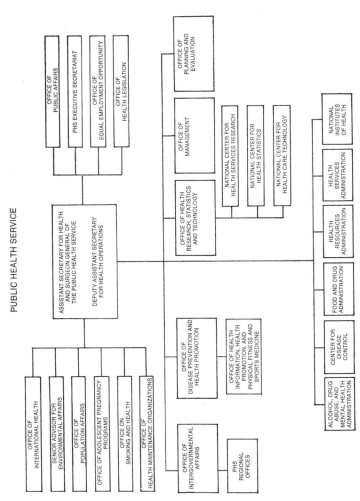

PUBLIC HEALTH SERVICE

Fig. 40. Department of Health and Human Services.

resulted in a continued downgrading of the role of the Public Health Service Commissioned Corps, and its replacement by a stronger Civil Service oriented "health component" of the Department of Health and Human Services in which the Service was previously housed.

The prominent role previously played by the Surgeon General of the Public Health Service has now been essentially taken over by the Assistant Secretary for Health who reports directly to the Secretary of the Department of Health and Human Services. Within the Assistant Secretary's office is lodged the responsibility for supervising all of the regional health administrators, who in turn function in each of 10 health regions into which the country has been divided. The regional health administrator and his staff are the representatives of the Assistant Secretary for Health in that region.

The Public Health Service is the federal agency charged by law to promote and assure the highest level of health attainable for every person in the United States and to develop cooperation in health programs with other nations. Its major functions are:

1. To stimulate and assist states and communities with the development of local health resources and to further the development of education for the health professions.

2. To assist with improvements in the delivery of health services to all Americans.

3. To conduct and support research in the medical and related sciences and to disseminate scientific information.

4. To protect the health of the Nation against unpure and unsafe foods, drugs and cosmetics, and other potential hazards.

5. To provide leadership for the prevention and control of communicable diseases.

The Public Health Service consists of six operating agencies with the Assistant Secretary for Health exercising direct line authority over these agencies.

Alcohol, Drug Abuse, and Mental Health Administration

The mission of this agency is to provide leadership in the federal effort to reduce, and where possible eliminate health problems caused by the abuse of alcohol and drugs and to improve the mental health of the people of the United States generally. It conducts and supports research, supports training of professional and paraprofessional personnel and supports service programs and projects including facilities construction. It collaborates with and provides technical assistance to state authorities and regional offices and supports state and community efforts in planning, establishing, maintaining and evaluating more effective programs. It also provides information on alcoholism, drug abuse and mental health to the public and to the scientific community.

Center for Disease Control

This is the federal agency charged with protecting the public health of the Nation by providing leadership and direction in the control of disease and other preventable conditions. It directs and enforces foreign quarantine activities and regulations and provides consultation and assistance in upgrading the performance of clinical laboratories. In order to assure safe and healthful working conditions, occupational safety and health standards are developed. It also provides consultation to other nations in the control of preventable diseases.

Food and Drug Administration

Its activities are directed toward protecting the health of the Nation against unpure and unsafe foods, drugs and cosmetics, and other potential hazards. It regulates biological products shipped in interstate and foreign commerce, develops policy with regard to safety, effectiveness, and labeling of all drugs for human use, develops standards on the composition, quality, nutrition and safety of foods and cosmetics, carries out programs designed to reduce exposure to hazardous radiation, develops policy regarding the safety, efficacy and labeling of medical devices and carries out research on the biological affects of potentially toxic chemical substances.

Health Resources Administration

This agency plans, develops and administers programs supporting the development and utilization of the Nation's health manpower and provides leadership and administration of areawide health planning and health delivery systems.

Health Services Administration

This agency helps communities find the best ways of meeting their health needs. It serves as a national focus in improving the organization and delivery of health care. It has particular concern for the development of health service delivery capacity for medically underserved areas and population groups and for the improvement of state or local systems of health care for mothers, children and adolescents. This agency operates a program of health services for eligible Indians and Alaskan Natives and provides health care services to designated federal beneficiaries through the Public Health Service hospital system. It also provides support to the U.S. Coast Guard.

National Institutes of Health

This agency conducts and supports biomedical research into the causes, prevention and cure of diseases, supports research training, and disseminates information to the scientific community. It actually consists of several separate institutions doing research on cancer, heart and lung diseases, arthritis, metabolism and digestive diseases, allergy and infectious diseases, child health and human development, dental health, environmental health, neurologic and communicable diseases, eye diseases, as well as an institute of general medical sciences and one on aging. The agency also operates a Clinical Center which is basically a hospital performing studies on specific diseases and disorders.

OTHER FEDERAL AGENCIES INVOLVED IN HEALTH

Also located within the Department of Health and Human Services is another agency which has major responsibilities in the field of medical care.

The Health Care Financing Administration

This entity was created in 1977 and places under one administration oversight of the Medicare and Medicaid programs which actually accounted in fiscal year 1978 for 80 per cent of the total Department of Health and Human Services expenditures for health. The agency also has responsibility for the related medical care quality control activities. It is concerned with the development of policies, procedures and guidance related to the Medicare program and is responsible for providing technical assistance to states and local organizations in regard to the Medicaid program. Its other responsibilities include implementation of the Professional Standards Review Organization's review activity as well as the end-stage renal disease program. Organizationally this agency responds directly to the Secretary of the Department of Health and Human Services.

Department of Labor

This Department has major responsibilities in occupational health and safety, and establishes standards for the protection of the worker.

Department of Agriculture

This Department has responsibility for inspection of meat and for the development of food supplement programs for low income families.

Department of Defense

This department has an extensive network of health facilities designed to provide medical care and health services to the military and their dependents.

Veterans Administration

This agency maintains a network of hospitals and clinics for the care of veterans.

HEALTH SERVICES AT THE STATE LEVEL

In the United States, each state has the responsibility for protection of the health of its citizens; the state is the sovereign power in this regard. The Federal Government possesses only those powers in the field of health delegated to it by the states. This is also true of local governments; their power and authority, too, are derived from the state.

Health laws in each of the states have considerable variation, but in all states there is provision for a Board of Health, or similar authority, whose responsibilities may be advisory but are often policy-making. The Board may also have the authority to enact regulations affecting the entire state, provided these are not inconsistent with state law.

Organization of health services at the State level, as with the Federal government, has undergone considerable change in the past few years. Essentially, the major change revolves around the growing tendency for the States to establish "umbrella agencies" such as a Department of Human Resources in which the health department as well as other departments such as welfare, mental hygiene and rehabilitation are included. The State Health Officer, in this case, reports to the Administrator of the umbrella agency rather than directly to the Governor.

The State Health Department is the agency vested by law with the responsibility for developing a variety of public health services that are aimed primarily at the protection of the health of citizens of the state. It also receives grants from the Federal Government which assist the state in developing health services. The type of health program carried on varies considerably within each state, but usually includes the compilation of vital statistics and the development of environmental health and public health laboratory services, communicable disease control, maternal and child health, public health nursing and health education. Many health departments, however, have much more extensive programs involving activities such as mental health and retardation, chronic disease services, accident prevention, medical care for the indigent and important licensing functions.

In order for the state health department to ensure adequate delivery of public health services throughout the state, various organizational patterns at the local level have been developed. While these differ with the states, they may, and often do, include the establishment of health departments at the county or city level. These local health departments, in turn, are responsible for providing services to the jurisdiction that they serve. Funds for the support of the state health department come primarily from state taxes, while those used to support local health departments emanate from local taxes, usually supported in varying degrees by state taxes.

One type of health organization that has, thus far, seen little growth in the United States is that based not upon a city or county but upon the metropolitan area. There are many good reasons which can be cited to support the desirability of organizing community health services on a metropolitan area basis. For example, the central city usually caters to an area which includes the adjoining suburbs for such items as shopping, work, and hospital and medical care. Certainly, air pollution control programs cannot be limited to just the central city. In spite of the many logical reasons that have been advanced for this type of health organization, its growth has been slow in this country, partially because of the political issues involved.

LOCAL HEALTH DEPARTMENTS

This century has seen radical population changes take place throughout the United States. There has been a strong tendency, particularly during the past 35 years, for the more affluent city dwellers to migrate to the suburbs, while the numbers of poorer persons who remain in the central part of the city have been swelled by migration from rural areas, particularly from the southern states. Further than this, the tendency has been not only for the central city to remain static or decrease in total population, but also for changes in the age distribution of that population to occur, resulting in an increasing number of children and older persons, with a concomitant drop in the age group 21 to 64, or, in other words, the wage earners.

These population changes have had a profound effect upon health departments, particularly those in metropolitan areas. Suburban health departments have grown in response to population increase, requiring services such as a potable water supply, sewage disposal, school health and mental health services. On the other hand, the large city health departments have been beset by tremendous problems resulting from the increase in children and senior citizens which has produced a growing demand for services. Thus, city health departments have in many cases had to develop extensive health services, including medical care services, for increasing numbers of economically deprived persons, unable to provide these services for themselves.

VOLUNTARY HEALTH AGENCIES

While no attempt is made here to describe all of these agencies, examples of a few of the better known ones follow:

National Council on Alcoholism

This was organized in 1944. It stimulates alcoholism programs through education and by devising methods to deal with industrial alcoholism. It fosters greater cooperation between labor and employee organizations in order to bring effective help to employees. It maintains a national resource materials center and carries on a program of professional education through workshops and conferences.

The Arthritis Foundation

Its objectives are the promotion and support of research, continuing education of physicians and allied health professionals, public education and demonstration programs and training support for community services and patient care functions.

Affiliated chapters provide funds for home-care programs, mobile units, visiting nurses and therapists, appliances, self-help devices and drugs.

The National Foundation—March of Dimes

Its mission is to organize and support programs of research, education, and services related to the causes and means of prevention and methods of treatment of birth defects. It has some 2,700 local chapters. Founded in 1938, this organization led the fight against poliomyelitis.

It provides grants to support both basic and clinical research related to birth defects and supplies informational material and supports professional education through conferences and teaching films. It also supports medical care programs through a network of birth defects centers which help provide care for patients with birth defects.

National Society for the Prevention of Blindness

This was organized in 1908 to find causes for blindness or impaired vision and to carry on activities for their prevention and for vision conservation through professional education, community services programs and research. It provided grants to hospitals and medical centers for eye disease research and sponsors professional conferences. It promotes individual eye safety programs as well as school and industrial eye safety programs and maintains an information and referral service.

American Cancer Society

This was organized in 1913 and provides grants for the support of studies on all aspects of cancer. It also conducts an intramural research program including large scale epidemologic studies. It carries out public educational activities and sponsors professional education, including a "Cancer Journal for Clinicians." It also conducts a service program to help and support the cancer patient and his family.

United Cerebral Palsy Associations

This organization maintains a research effort relating to cerebral palsy but studies prematurity, obstetrical and parental factors, neurotropic viruses and hyperbilirubinemia of the newborn. It also operates a small grants program, carries on professional and educational activities and allocates almost two-thirds of its funds for patient services through state and local affiliates.

American Diabetes Association

This organization supports research and development awards given to young promising scientists, grants for research in any phase of diabetes primarily necessary to provide equipment and an annual series of symposia. It carries on public education through the use of case finding and provides diabetes testing kits and agents which are distributed by its local and state affiliates each year. It carries on professional education and publishes a scientific journal "Diabetes" and publishes a variety of patient oriented material, including a cook book for diabetics.

Epilepsy Foundation of America

Its objectives are to institute programs in finding answers to the problems of epilepsy and to bring about the successful integration of epileptics into society. Research, education, and service programs addressing special medical, economic, and social gaps have been instituted by this organization. It also publishes literature dealing with legal rights of persons with epilepsy and has established an information, travel, and referral service.

National Easter Seal Society for Crippled Children and Adults

This organization provides rehabilitation services to alleviate the physical, psychologic, social and vocational effects of crippling diseases or injury. It performs these services primarily through its affiliates which operate a number of evaluation and treatment centers, rehabilitation centers, speech programs, workshops, activities for home bound persons, and recreational programs. Braces and appliances are also provided, equipment loaned, and transportation provided. The organization also maintains a public and professional education program and sponsors research projects at universities and medical centers throughout the country.

American Heart Association

This organization supports postdoctoral research in cardiovascular disease and its affiliates provide support to postgraduate fellowship and research projects. The organization carries on a public education and an extensive professional education program as well as individual training courses in cardiopulmonary resuscitation. Its affiliates sponsor programs including rehabilitation, workshops, visits, and vocational guidance. They also encourage and assist in the development of coronary care units in community hospitals.

National Kidney Foundation

This organization has as its primary objective the promotion of the care and treatment of kidney disease both in hospitals and in the community. It supports basic and clinical research, promotes professional and public education, awards fellowships, and grants to those qualified in order to encourage advanced training in the care of patients with kidney disease and supports direct care services programs to establish drug banks to provide needed medicine at the lowest possible cost.

Planned Parenthood—Life and World Population

The major purpose of this organization is to provide leadership in making effective means of voluntary fertility control fully accessible to all. It also stimulates relevant biomedical, socioeconomic and demographic research, maintains public and professional educational activities, and helps develop liaison between public and private organizations in developing family planning services.

National Association for Mental Health

Its purpose is to develop a coordinated citizen's movement to work toward care and treatment of the mentally ill and handicapped, to improve methods in providing services, diagnosis and treatment to the mentally ill and to promote mental health. Its main research has been in the area of schizophrenia.

National Association for Retarded Children

This organization is devoted to promoting the welfare of the mentally retarded of all ages. It supports a wide variety of reading programs and research into mental retardation. It helps encourage the development of rehabilitation programs and provides vocational training and work experience which will assist the retard to live independently in the community.

National Tuberculosis and Respiratory Diseases Association

Founded in 1904, this organization is now engaged in a campaign to control such diseases as chronic bronchitis, emphysema and asthma, as well as tuberculosis. It supports research projects, carries on public and professional education, and its affiliates assist in identifying the need for screening, diagnostic, treatment, and rehabilitation services.

The American National Red Cross

This organization assists in carrying out the obligation assumed by the United States under a number of international treaties by which it carries on national and international activities to alleviate the sufferng caused by disaster.

The Red Cross maintains a blood program consisting of regular blood centers which collect blood from voluntary donors. It also maintains a number of safety programs including courses in first aid, craft, and water safety. Red Cross volunteers also serve in hospitals, nursing homes and other institutions. There are some 3,300 Red Cross chapters across the United States.

REFERENCES

AMA Directory of National Voluntary Health Organizations, Chicago, Illinois, 1971.

The National Health Council, Voluntaryism and Health, New York, 1962.

Rosen, G.: *A History of Public Health*, New York, M. D. Publications, Inc., 1958.

Stebbins, E. L.: International Health Organization, in Sartwell *Preventive Medicine and Public Health*, Maxcy and Rosenau (Eds.), 10th Ed., New York, Appleton-Century-Crofts, 1973.

U.S. Government Manual, Washington, D.C., 1978–79.

Index